THERE IS NOTHING SUPERNATURAL ABOUT THE "MIRACLE CURES" THE BODY CAN ACHIEVE

This book will tell you:

—How the different organs of the body are geared to combat anything that interferes with the body's proper functioning.

—How antibodies and other substances that the body produces deal with germs, viruses, heart diseases, and even cancer cells.

—How vitamins, proper diet, exercise, relaxation, and other easily mastered self-help programs work to strengthen the body's defense mechanisms.

—How nature means for you to be healthy and to stay healthy, and how you can be as healthy as you were meant to be.

THE DOCTOR WITHIN

THE DOCTOR WITHIN

by Hal Zina Bennett

Foreword by Lendon Smith, M.D.

Illustrations by Bill Wells

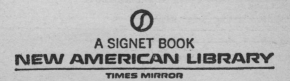

A SIGNET BOOK

NEW AMERICAN LIBRARY

TIMES MIRROR

PUBLISHER'S NOTE

The ideas, procedures, and suggestions contained in this book are not intended as a substitute for consulting with your physician. All matters regarding your health require medical supervision.

NAL BOOKS ARE AVAILABLE AT QUANTITY DISCOUNTS WHEN USED TO PROMOTE PRODUCTS OR SERVICES. FOR INFORMATION PLEASE WRITE TO PREMIUM MARKETING DIVISION, THE NEW AMERICAN LIBRARY, INC., 1633 BROADWAY, NEW YORK, NEW YORK 10019.

Special thanks to Nancy Novogrod and Carolyn Hart

Published by arrangement with Clarkson N. Potter, Inc. The original edition was published simultaneously in Canada by General Publishing Company Limited.

SIGNET, SIGNET CLASSICS, MENTOR, PLUME, MERIDIAN AND NAL BOOKS are published by The New American Library, Inc., 1633 Broadway, New York, New York 10019

First Signet Printing, July, 1982

1   2   3   4   5   6   7   8   9

PRINTED IN THE UNITED STATES OF AMERICA

Dedicated to
Martha Evenson Bennett, my mother,
who planted the seeds for many ideas
that have come to fruition here

Contents

Foreword

This cheerful and encouraging book provides a sound program for the care and maintenance of the human body and mind. It makes good health sound invitingly easy to achieve. All you need is relaxation, exercise, optimum nutrition, and the belief that your well-being is within your control.

As a medical doctor, I was trained to believe that physicians alone hold all the keys to good health. We could prescribe medicines and surgery. We could rely on X ray for diagnosis and therapy. If we were stumped, we could pack the patient off to the laboratory for blood and urine tests, and if these failed to reveal the problem, we could suggest a psychiatrist to treat the symptoms. If someone got sick too often, we suspected he had bad genes or poor protoplasm.

In my pediatrics practice over the past thirty years, the parents of my patients have often asked me why their children were continually sick. They had been fed, bathed, and loved. Why weren't they protected from illness? Until recently, my response was always inadequate: "It's a phase"; "Lots of kids are like that"; or "Everyone gets sick."

In the last ten years I have been searching for better answers. I have experimented with many of the approaches this book describes. And they work. My personal interest is in vitamins and nutrition, and I've been fascinated by the health benefits that can be achieved from this modality alone.

Some doctors of medicine would insist that the remedies Hal Bennett suggests are unproven at best and blatant quackery at worst. The traditional medical approach to disease has been to make a diagnosis and prescribe a treatment. No thought at all was given to why the patient originally got sick. What slipped? What stress factor or food deficiency, for example, may have lowered the immune system to the point where a virus infection could get inside the cells? Patients today are seeking more knowledge of how their bodies work and demanding that their physicians take a closer look at the underlying causes of illness and disease.

Without resorting to accusations aimed at the medical profession, Mr. Bennett calmly and cogently explains how we can all have a greater chance for a healthier, and maybe even a longer, life if we follow the proven paths he lays out for us.

As a matter of fact, doctors would do themselves and their patients a service by sending out this book with their bills.

LENDON SMITH, M.D.
January 1981

A NOTE ABOUT TOOL KITS

This book contains detailed instructions for specific measures you can take to strengthen your resistance to disease. The symbol of a physician's little black bag identifies the passages that describe self-care tools. Taken together, the tool kits constitute a program for building optimal resistance to disease. You can tailor them to your own needs. For easy reference, I have provided the following complete list of tool kits and the page numbers in which they appear:

Introduction

THE VIRUS THAT CAUSED your last cold didn't go away because it got tired of your company. On the contrary, it was annihilated by aggressive actions taken by your body's doctor within. Far from being a passive victim to disease, the human body rallies its healing forces and removes the offender or repairs damaged tissue with as much vigor as the world's best-trained medical team.

Our knowledge of the human body's self-healing powers has been expanded tremendously by medical science in recent years, and, ironically, this new, commonsense appreciation for what I call "the doctor within" has caused many physicians to reassess medical techniques that were previously accepted forms of treatment. In the medical community, and among lay people, there is a growing belief that we all may have been overawed by the inventions of medical technology, inventions such as antibiotics and vaccination and, more recently, open-heart surgery. We are beginning to recognize that we were too hasty in giving medicine credit for mastering disease and, what's more important, that we have allowed our misplaced trust in modern medicine to overshadow the more powerful and ultimately more important healing capacities we each have within our own bodies.

We are at a happy turning point in medical history, when, having recognized the outer limits of technological medicine, doctors and lay people are together discovering the vast powers for creating health that we inherit at birth. The reaffirmation of those powers is nowhere better realized than in the self-help health movement, a movement that is significantly changing American medicine.

Most people practice self-help health at least on some level. It may mean going down to the drugstore for aspirin or vitamin C when you feel a cold coming on, or cutting down on the intake of eggs and animal fats to reduce your cholesterol count. On a more aggressive level it may mean getting started on a regular exercise program to tone up your cardiovascular system. We know that the actions we take along these lines improve our own lives, and for most of us that's enough. Looking beyond that, however, you might be startled to see that these actions are changing the ways American medicine is being practiced. There are those in the medical professions who believe that this trend toward self-help health is bringing new knowledge to modern medicine that is at least as profound as the discovery of penicillin in the 1940s or the beginning of smallpox vaccination at the turn of the century.

A Remedy for the Aches and Pains of Everyday Life

Self-help health is a system of medicine addressed not to rare diseases treatable in hospitals but to the aches and pains of everyday life, treatable at home. Its central philosophy grows out of medical research and clinical observation borrowed from mainstream medicine, experience that indicates that many serious diseases can be avoided by treating the minor ones. The belief is that your aches and pains are important messages from your body, telling you to do something, to change something in your life so that you'll be more comfortable.

Many of the principles of self-help health are simply common sense, one of the most obvious and, at the same time, important health tools we possess. For example, change what you're eating when you have simple indigestion day after day. And seek ways to relax or to use your body in a better way when you have headaches three times a week. And ease into a physical exercise program when you see yourself becoming flabby, your energy waning, and vague "bone pains" creeping in.

The self-help health movement has been responsible for at least two great contributions to modern medicine: (1) making medical information accessible to nonmedical people, and (2) inventing tools and techniques that people can apply for themselves.

Before self-help gained impetus, the medical community was well aware of the shortcomings of crisis-oriented medicine. One of the greatest shortcomings was that doctors were at a complete loss about what to do for many of the people who came to their offices. Though suffering, these people had nothing that could be cured by the drugs and surgical procedures, which were the main tools of the modern physician. Furthermore, physicians knew, as the old saying goes, that "an ounce of prevention is worth a pound of cure." They knew that many of the untreatable complaints would ultimately become treatable: The tense person with chronic indigestion would eventually turn up with a bleeding ulcer; the smoker with chronic headaches would eventually turn up with high blood pressure—or worse; the slightly overweight, listless housewife who complained of bone pain would eventually turn up with arthritis. Except for vaccines for a handful of infectious diseases, the modern physician had virtually no prevention tools.

Where Modern Medicine Has Failed

In spite of our advanced technological approach to healing, some startling recent revelations indicate that modern medicine has done surprisingly little to improve the nation's health. These findings show that the incidence of disease is as high as ever (higher in a few cases), even though some of the *kinds* of diseases have changed. Although American medicine has improved in the *treatment* of diseases already contracted, it has done surprisingly little to *prevent* those diseases from occurring in the first place. Moreover, the cost of treating diseases has risen to $206 billion annually, or a staggering 9.1 percent of our gross national product!

One of the measurements used to evaluate a nation's health system is the infant mortality rate, since normal births are so positively affected by prenatal care, proper nutrition, and the health knowledge of the mother. If this is in fact true, we in the United States have a lot of room for improvement. A revealing study published by the United Nations compared figures on the seventeen most technologically advanced countries of the world, countries with medical systems comparable to our own. Of those seventeen, the United States had the *highest infant mortality rate*. That is, we had more infant deaths per pregnancy than any of the other sixteen nations.

Among the most alarming developments in modern medicine is the rising incidence of *iatrogenic* disease—that is, disease caused by medical treatment. There was a time when wars, nature, and one's own negligence were the major causes of suffering and death. But because of the size and intricacy of the science of medicine, the power of procedures employed by physicians, and the extent of involvement of the medical establishment in our lives, medical treatment has taken its place alongside these other natural and man-made disasters. Malpractice may contribute to the statistics for this disease, but, for the most part, iatrogenic disease is caused by treatment administered in a medically acceptable way.

It would be comforting to believe that even though modern medicine cannot always promise a cure, its remedies at least are benign. But the facts don't support us in this. Let me cite a few examples:

Example: A study done by Dr. N. S. Iney for the Armed Forces Institute of Pathology estimates that there are somewhere between 6,000 and 12,000 deaths each year caused by reactions to drugs prescribed in the treatment of disease.

Example: In a book called *How to Avoid Unnecessary Surgery*,* the author, Laurence P. Williams, himself a surgeon, estimates that unnecessary surgery may kill as many as 10,000 people each year. The subtitle of one medical report speaks for itself: "A Study Based on Removal of 704 Normal Ovaries from 546 Patients." Another study, based on 6,960 cases, showed that examinations by pathologists following surgery established *at least some* justification for the removal of ovaries in *only slightly more than half the cases!*

Example: According to figures published by the National Center for Health Statistics, tonsillectomy is the most common surgical procedure performed in Western civilization. But, according to Dr. A. Frederick North, Jr., Visiting Professor of Pediatrics at the University of Pittsburgh, 90 to 95 percent of these operations are completely unnecessary. Furthermore, there is evidence that the removal of the tonsils (1) reduces the effectiveness of a person's immune system for the rest of his or her life; (2) may be linked to an increased risk of contracting Hodgkin's disease; and (3) increases the risk of bulbar poliomyelitis. The surgical procedure itself causes an estimated 100 to 300 deaths each year, and in more than 15 cases per 1,000 there are serious medical complications.

Example: One out of every five people admitted to research hospitals for medical care acquires a disease caused by the treatment they receive. Of these, one in thirty results in death. One in ten of these occurs as the result of a diagnostic procedure.

Example: Infections contracted in hospitals exceed the rate contracted in the average household! Hospital infections, by the way, can be extremely serious, since certain bacteria have evolved new forms and new characteristics within the hospital environment and have become resistant to antibiotics. One of the most serious infections of this kind is caused by resistant strains of gram-negative bacteria. A report in *Annals of Internal*

---

* Laurence P. Williams, *How to Avoid Unnecessary Surgery* (New York: Warner Paperback Library, 1972).

Medicine warns physicians that gram-negative bacteria may be killing as many as 100,000 people each year! Because gram-negative infections are so common, the evolution of strains that are resistant to antibiotics is quite a serious issue.

Example: The frequency of reported accidents in hospitals is higher than in any other industrial site except mines and high-rise steel construction.

Noting these and other problems in our medical system, Ivan Illich, in his book *Medical Nemesis,** reflected that:

The pain, dysfunction, disability, and anguish resulting from technical medical intervention now rival the morbidity due to traffic and industrial accidents and even war-related activities, and make the impact of medicine one of the most rapidly spreading epidemics of our time.

The Healing Powers of Your Doctor Within

Whereas a knowledge of disease is the foundation of traditional medicine, a knowledge of health is the foundation of the self-help health movement. In the latter, knowledge begins with what I am calling the doctor within, that network of healing systems we each possess within our body.

The doctor within is both a figurehead and a reality. As a figurehead, it reminds us that health is created from the inside and is the product of our own efforts. It reminds us that individual powers exceed those of institutions. Interestingly enough, the *reality* is the same as the figurehead; that is, health really is created from within, maintained from moment to moment by mental and physiological processes, some of which are very simple, some of which are so sophisticated they elude scientific scrutiny.

Often, the processes of the doctor within exhibit a kind of beauty, a concert of events as perfect as the mysterious order of our galaxy. There is beauty, for example, in the step-by-step chemical process the human body goes through to repair

---

* Ivan Illich, *Medical Nemesis* (New York: Pantheon, 1976).

a cut finger or restore a broken bone. Similarly, one is amazed by the processes of analysis and synthesis the doctor within calls upon to identify a bacterium or virus and create chemicals to neutralize it. And then there are the biofeedback systems throughout your body that direct the life processes such as blood flow, muscle tension, hormonal secretions, and body temperature to meet the changing demands of your body as you go through the normal events of a day.

As you acquaint yourself with your inner resources, and you discover their vast powers as well as their limits, subjects such as diet, exercise, and stress reduction will take on new meaning. For example, you will see how blood vessels are strengthened, expanded, and cleansed after physical exercise, aiding in the delivery of nutrients and antibodies and hormones to all areas of your body. Suddenly, apparently faddish diets, the jogging craze, and myriad other health-related regimens that have been thrust upon the public in recent years begin to seem worthy of new respect.

As the mysteries of the doctor within unfold to you, your response will be relief and awe—relief to discover that you are not, after all, prey to disease, and awe at the power you hold within you. You will see very clearly that your healing and regenerative functions have the same down-to-earth reality as your skin, muscles, bones, hair, and fingernails. As you assimilate this new knowledge, your doctor within should become a source of security that will be with you throughout your life.

As your familiarity with your inner healing system grows, the skills of the doctor within become your own skills, just as the skills of reading, writing, or driving a car become yours. At that point you begin to change in your thinking; your knowledge of your doctor within transports you from the role of passive victim when you are sick to the role of a very active and skillful healer.

1.

The Inner Ecology of Disease Resistance

BEFORE YOU WERE BORN you shared your mother's immunity system. You were protected from the same diseases for which she had developed immunities in her lifetime. This becomes obvious, of course, when you realize that in your earliest days you were nurtured by the same fluids of her body that nurtured her own organs and muscle tissue, fluids that carried all the stuff of immunity. Until you left her body your immunity status was the same as that of any one of her vital organs.

Your thymus gland, in your fetal period, was the brain and memory of your developing immunity system. It is as though the doctor within uses the thymus gland to store the information he learns from your mother's body and from her experience with maintaining health. Your thymus gland received and stored all this knowledge, and later it learned to create its own antibodies capable of protecting you from disease.

If you were breast-fed by your mother, her defenses continued to protect you after birth. Antibodies produced by your mother's doctor within were transferred directly to you through your mother's milk. These antibodies helped you combat a wide variety of disease-causing bacteria. Breast-fed babies have been found to have fewer respiratory tract infections, a lower incidence of meningitis, and generally a greater resistance to viral infections than babies who have been bottle-fed on formula.* And the benefits of breast-feeding last through life—even the incidence of a disease associated with old age, arteriosclerosis, arising from a buildup of fats in the arteries, has been found to be lower in people who were breast-fed.

The dozens of diseases you were subjected to as a child contributed more antibody knowledge to your doctor within. Within a young child's peer group there is the richest pool of disease organisms in the world. In the medical community it is now generally agreed that this early experience with minor infections is healthy. With each new infection, new configurations of antibodies are synthesized, building up a vast library for the doctor within to draw upon. This library was enriched even further by the vaccinations you received as a child.

Several years ago there was a television film made about a young boy whose immunity system didn't work. Of course, without this system he would have died within a matter of a few hours of his birth, his death caused by viruses or bacteria that you or I, with our fully functioning immunity systems, would easily have shrugged off. To save the child, doctors encased him in a plastic bubble, which, like a space suit, created a sterile environment, free of disease-causing microorganisms his body had no tools to combat. The image of a person living inside a plastic bubble dramatically symbolizes the tremendous service our immunity system provides.

Self and Not-Self: The Essential Issues for Immunity

For the doctor within, the issues of immunity are simplified down to a single concept. That concept is this: Where the human body is concerned, there are only two classifications of

---

* Mike Samuels and Nancy Samuels, *The Well Baby Book* (New York: Summit Books, 1979).

substances or organisms possible. Each must be either *self* or *not-self*. That which is self must be protected. That which is not-self must be destroyed.

This directive, however, is more complicated than it sounds. The fact is that many bacteria, even some that are known to cause disease, actually live on our skin and within our bodies. These bacteria not only are tolerated but are encouraged by the doctor within.

It had been found, for example, that upward of fifteen different types of bacteria and viruses normally live in our mouths and upper respiratory tracts. These normal inhabitants include pneumococcal and streptococcal bacteria, families of microbes that can, under certain circumstances, cause pneumonia, bronchitis, and strep throat infections. Similarly, most people's noses contain adenoviruses, a strain of viruses sometimes implicated in upper respiratory infections. These viruses have even been found in the noses of babies only seconds after birth.

Once the bacteria and viruses normal to these areas establish residence there, they protect their territory, just as animals in the wild do. After all, there is only so much space for them and only a limited food supply. If they are to live harmoniously with other microbes, they must work together to keep foreigners out.

Microbial Ecosystems

In recent years we've all become increasingly aware of the science of ecology, that is, of our dependence on the delicate balances that exist among ourselves, the lower animals, plants, insects, earth, water, air, and the microbial world. Each human action, regardless of our intentions, changes the course of life around us, sometimes for better, sometimes for worse.

Although we are now familiar with the workings of the ecosystems in the environment, most people have only scratched the surface when it comes to understanding the ecosystems of their own bodies. These ecosystems operate with the same complex dynamics of the larger ecosystems in nature.

For the sake of clarification, let's try to draw some simple parallels between the relationships within our bodies and the environment of a marsh pond. Every species of animal, insect, mold, alga, bacterium, and vegetation in and around the pond is essential to it. If you take away any one of its parts the total system may be threatened. Take away the insects, and the fish and reptiles, deprived of an important element of their food chain, die out. Once the fish that are their source of food are gone, the ducks will no longer nest there. Algae, normally part of the food chain of ducks and some reptiles, begin reproducing wildly, no longer held in check by the higher species. The algae clogs the water of the pond. The pond putrifies and, in effect, dies, unable to support the complex community of life forms that once lived there.

These same dynamics exist in our own bodies. The entity whom you think of as you is not composed of a single type of organism. You, like the marsh pond, are a complex system with many microorganisms living in and on you. The mutually beneficial relationships of these microorganisms have evolved over millions of years. Each microorganism has a role, a purpose for living. Some of them produce nutrients that your doctor within uses to heal damaged tissue—which we'll be discussing in a moment. Others are scavengers, eating bacteria or the waste products of bacteria, that might otherwise cause you harm. Some guard you, producing substances that repel foreign bacteria that might otherwise cause disease. And some, just like the algae in the marsh pond, appear to have no purpose other than to provide food for bacteria.

As a general rule, the microbes within an ecosystem are highly specialized. They have exacting environmental needs. If the food supplies, temperature, acid-base, or moisture levels of their place of residence are off even a small amount, or if the other organisms with which they normally live aren't present in sufficient number, they can't survive. As long as their surroundings conform to their exact needs they are strong, healthy, and productive members of a larger ecosystem.

In the study of ecology one learns to respect every participant within an ecosystem. The same principles that apply to the marsh pond apply to our bodies. *Escherichia coli* bacteria, for example, live productive and beneficial lives in our intestines. But if allowed to invade outer skin surfaces they could become the agents of disease. Millions of these *E. coli* bacteria pass out of the intestines, carried in the feces, in the normal daily process of elimination. The *E. coli* would cause serious infection except for the fact that adjacent skin surfaces are protected by a family of bacteria classified as scavengers because they survive on waste substances. These scavenger bacteria, which are nourished by what is essentially waste *E. coli*, live harmoniously with the microbes in their community on the surface of the skin.

Thus we begin to understand that bacteria and other microorganisms that we might under certain circumstances identify as foreign invaders are participating in a larger plan designed to keep us healthy. The bacteria that stake out our skin are an excellent example of the protective functions of microbes.

Every day our skin comes in contact with millions of bacteria and viruses in the environment. What prevents foreign bacteria from taking up residence there is that our skin is already staked out by the bacterial strain known as staphylococcus. These bacteria, which normally live in total harmony with us, are members of a community of microbes that keep foreign invaders out. As far as scientists have been able to tell, staphylococci that live on our skin have no other function or purpose than to protect their community from not-self substances. They discourage foreign bacteria by secreting substances that are toxic to the would-be invaders. Sometimes these bacteria simply crowd out the foreigners, proliferating at a rate that makes it impossible for the outsiders to compete for space. And sometimes our territory-guarding microbes eliminate the outsiders simply by eating them.

Territory-guarding bacteria generally do their work in two ways: first, by maintaining, through their own secretions, an environment of a particular acid level that is pleasant for helpful bacteria but noxious to others; second, by producing and secreting substances that work like poisons to destroy microbes that might otherwise be harmful to the host.

One of the most interesting examples of protection by an acid environment takes place in the vagina. At birth and until a girl approaches adolescence, the normal moist secretions of her vagina's mucous membranes are slightly on the alkaline side. During this early period of life her vagina harbors only a sparse population of microbes. As adolescence approaches, the mucus of the vagina changes. Vaginal membranes begin producing glycogen along with the normal secretions, largely as a result of sex hormones that develop at this time. New bacteria appear, notably Döderlein bacilli and yeast. These microorganisms are the doctor within's choices for protecting this orifice. Döderlein bacilli ferment the glycogen in the normal vaginal secretions, causing the environment to change from an alkaline to an acid one.

After the acid environment is established it can be seen as a tool of the doctor within. It acts to exclude more microbes that can cause infection, which are likely to be introduced when menstruation, sexual activity, and childbirth occur. This environment must be sufficiently strong to resist or to accept and live harmoniously with the microbes that the male brings to the vagina during intercourse.

A very complex and powerful environmental dynamic takes place. The vagina's microbial ecosystem must be dependable and strong to protect the organs of reproduction from infection, a task that is essential to preserving the human species.

At first glance the state of balance in the microbial ecosystems of our bodies would seem tenuous at best. But the truth is these balances are extremely stable and strong. They resist negative influences very well indeed.

The Mucosal Blanket

The main channels into your body, that is, your mouth and nose, need special protection, since it is through these orifices that substances ranging from the tiniest virus to the heaviest industrial pollutants may pass. Solving the problem of how to allow air and food to enter while keeping out potentially harmful substances requires some extraordinary efforts on the part of your doctor within.

The mucosal blanket is a constantly moving river of mucus that lines your nose, throat, and trachea, which form the passages to your lungs. It works much like a conveyor belt. Particles tossed onto it are carried to the back of your throat. Some particles are then exhaled, coughed, or sneezed back into the air. Others are conveyed down the passage to your stomach, where acids normal to digestion dissolve them, rendering them harmless to your health. In the fluid river created by the mucosal blanket there is a complex ecosystem of bacteria and viruses that live in perfect harmony with one another as well as with your tissue cells, protecting you from foreign invaders.

Gravity, along with the constant production of mucus by cells in your nose and sinuses, moves the blanket from around your pharynx (the back of your throat) down to that area. Cilia, that is, microscopic hairs, constantly waving along the air passages to your lungs, keep the mucosal blanket moving uphill, from your lungs toward your pharynx. The mucosal blanket moves at the rate of about two feet per hour, a significant speed when you consider the relatively short distance it travels.

As air moves into your nostrils, the hairs lining them filter out the larger particles, trapping them in the mucus in the vestibule of your nose. Smaller particles are bounced around by the turbulent air that moves through the various twists and turns of your nasal passages. In the process of being bounced around, microscopic particles become trapped in the sticky mucus. Substances in the mucus can, by themselves, dissolve and digest a number of foreign particles, ranging from house dust to certain kinds of viruses.

Occasionally, particles that might be harmful to you make their way past your nasal passages and mouth into your trachea. But here, too, they encounter the mucosal blanket. Mucus in your trachea picks up foreign particles before they can reach your bronchial tubes or your lungs. Once in your lungs, they might otherwise lodge in your microscopic alveoli and cause serious disease. Thanks to the mucosal blanket, this seldom happens. Particles picked up in your trachea are shunted up to the area at the back of your throat, powered upward, and expelled by your cilia.

One reason cigarette smoking is harmful to your health is that particles in the smoke are too small to be picked up by the mucosal blanket. Thus, these tiniest of all particles make their way to your lungs, and do, in fact, lodge in the alveoli.

Trapped in the alveoli, these particles are surrounded and chewed up by white blood cells. But if you are a moderate to heavy smoker the white blood cells can't keep up with the amount of smoke you're drawing into your lungs. The particles that escape being cleaned out by white blood cells cause the growth of fibrous tissue, contributing heavily to diseases such as emphysema and cancer. In addition, the nicotine paralyzes cilia in your trachea, slowing down or even stopping the flow of your mucosal blanket.

Your mucosal blanket is also responsible for humidifying the air you breathe. If air is too dry before it enters your lungs, it can dry out the tissue, causing it to become raw or cracked, just as can happen to your lips in dry climates, and the raw tissue then becomes highly susceptible to infection.

In the past decade or so, medical researchers have discovered a correlation between an increase in colds, especially summer colds, and air conditioning. More people than ever work and live in buildings that are "climate controlled" by central air-conditioning plants. In most commercial buildings constructed since the early 1950s, it is not even possible to open windows to get fresh air. Except for a few air-conditioning systems that also humidify the air, central air conditioning dries out the mucosal blanket and makes people vulnerable to infections from which they would otherwise be well protected.

The Bacterial Garden in Our Intestines

In the process of healing cuts and breaks, the doctor within sends a substance called prothrombin to the area that needs mending. This prothrombin, a protein, bridges the wound and begins the healing. Without a micronutrient called vitamin K, prothrombin could not be produced, and the wound would never be healed. Most vitamin K used in the production of prothrombin comes not from the foods we eat but from a garden of bacteria inside our intestines.

In addition to cultivating bacteria that supply vitamin K, the doctor within cultivates bacteria in the intestinal garden that supply us with an endless source of the essential B vitamins, notably B_{12}, without which life itself would not be possible. Our bodies use the B vitamins for creating DNA, the genetic material of every cell. In addition, B_{12} plays an important role in the maturation of red blood cells, produced in our bone marrow. Immature red blood cells, deprived of B_{12}, become oversized, fewer in number, and have reduced capacity for transporting oxygen, one of their essential tasks in our bodies. B vitamins also aid in the regeneration of tissues throughout our bodies. The doctor within uses this micronutrient group for producing antibodies to fight infections. In the area of digestion, without B vitamins we could not fully metabolize fats and carbohydrates.

According to Bernard Dixon, in his book *Magnificent Microbes*,* there is still another use, recently discovered, for bacteria in our intestines. This is one that will please people who eat a lot of refined foods. Bacteria in our intestines have been found to be effective in breaking down food additives. Without the intervention of these bacteria, chemicals added to food to provide color and flavor might otherwise become carcinogenic.

Interestingly enough, our knowledge of how microbes living in our intestines keep us well came to light as a result of modern drug therapies. As antibiotics came into popular use, certain diseases began to appear in people who relied too frequently on these drugs. If your doctor within is unable to get hold of the B vitamins, these diseases can result. They include pernicious anemia, psychiatric disturbances such as chronic irritability and lack of concentration ability, and even spinal lesions. Chronic indigestion also plagues antibiotic users. While destroying bacteria that are causing infections, the drugs are also destroying the bacterial gardens so carefully cultivated by the doctor within.

How Microbes Keep Us Well

In light of these scientific insights into microbes and microbial ecosystems, we must considerably extend our vision of the microbial world. Of the thousands of species of microbes that exist, only a few hundred species cause serious human

* Bernard Dixon, *Magnificent Microbes* (New York: Atheneum Books, 1979).

disease. The overwhelming majority of them are beneficial. The fact is, our lives would be absolutely impossible without them.

Perhaps because we are now relatively free of the kinds of anxieties we once had about infectious disease, we can afford to take this broader view. It is now recognized that microbes benefit human life in many different ways, from teaching our immunity systems to develop rich storehouses of antibody knowledge, to nitrogen-fixing via the plants we eat, to the culturing and fermenting of cheese and wine products.

One of the best indicators we have that we are expanding our understanding of microbes is found in the growing science of "gnotobiology": the study of the relationships that exist between animals, such as ourselves, and microbes. Research in this field has shown that animals raised in germ-free environments become extremely vulnerable to infections that animals raised in normal environments tolerate easily.

It is believed—and at least partially proved—that the animal raised in environments devoid of microbes never develops its immunity system fully. It is as though the sterile environment deprives the immune system of essential antibody-building experience. When introduced to a normal, nonsterile environment, disease and death come quickly to animals deprived in this way; they simply don't have the antibodies to combat even low levels of infection. These animals manifest other more unexpected anomalies. They develop defects in their intestinal tract structures and unusual nutritional requirements, especially in the B vitamin group. And what is most surprising is that even their heart activity is weaker than normal.

Recent experiments with microbes have taken our knowledge of bacteria still further. Scientists are attempting to use bacteria to stimulate the normal internal healing processes of the doctor within.

In Quebec, Canada, medical researchers observed a decreased incidence of leukemia in children immunized with *Bacillus Calmette-Guérin* (BCG). This is a live bacterium related to the microbe that causes tuberculosis. It is routinely given to schoolchildren in Quebec to protect them from tuberculosis. Is there any direct correlation between these immunizations and the low incidence of childhood leukemia?

The evidence would certainly seem to indicate that. There have been reports of limited but clinically promising success in treating leukemia victims with BCG after they were diagnosed as having this form of cancer.

BCG has also been injected into laboratory animals with malignant tumors. That it effectively reduced those tumors in most cases is less startling than it sounds.

BACTERIA AS A CURE FOR CANCER

Over the years physicians have observed relationships between bacterial infections and spontaneous remissions of cancer. In the nineteenth century, an English doctor by the name of Coley stood by the bedside of a patient dying of cancer. The patient got worse each day. When the physician discovered the dying man was developing a serious bacterial infection in the same area as his cancer, he believed the end was in sight. However, the tumor suddenly began to shrink. Miraculously, the patient got increasingly better until he had achieved total recovery from both the cancer and the bacterial infection.

In a great number of documented cases, malignant tumors have disappeared after the patient contracted a serious bacterial infection. Researchers have demonstrated that the immune response is less likely to be stimulated by cancer than by bacteria. Unless the host is feeble and malnourished, bacteria seldom fail to rally the full force of the immunity system. In cases of spontaneous remission of cancer, bacteria are given credit for mobilizing immune mechanisms so that they go after not only the bacteria but the cancer as well.

There is still much to be learned about this field of medicine, but the outlook is promising. Researchers are hoping to develop bacteria that while not capable of causing infections of their own will have the capacity to make the immune system rally against cancer.

Antibiotics: Helpful or Harmful?

Although the practice is less prevalent now than it was a few years ago, doctors still prescribe antibiotics without concern for the personal ecosystem of the patient. For example, few physicians ever explain to their patients that the normal bacteria that live in and on you, and that are actually healing instruments of your doctor within, are threatened by antibiotics. I do not want to sound like an alarmist here, yet I do want the point to be clear. *Whenever you take antibiotics, the microbial ecosystems that are necessary to your health are going to be disrupted*, just as assuredly as destroying all the mosquitoes in a marsh is going to disrupt that ecosystem.

It should be common knowledge, but unfortunately it's not, that when a woman is given an antibiotic for, let's say, a strep throat infection, it is not unusual for that treatment to be followed by a vaginal infection. The reason for this is quite simple. The antibiotic for the strep infection will act upon all bacteria in her body. The normal bacteria of her vagina are destroyed along with the strep, leaving the normal yeast of that area free to reproduce wildly. The infection that follows, caused by the yeast, can be controlled by Nystatin, a drug that both kills and prevents the replication of yeasts. After taking this drug to correct the problem created by taking the other drug, your doctor within eventually gets back to the business of restoring the normal balance of your bacterial ecosystems. But all of that takes time.

Bacteria, like all other organisms in the universe, are just trying to get along. It may be difficult to find sympathy for them, especially when they're implicated in a disease you're suffering from, but that sympathy is essential for understanding your interactions with them. Like the rest of us on this planet, each microbe has a defense mechanism, a doctor within, if you will, whose job it is to keep the species alive—that is, to protect it from harmful entities in its environment.

The traits of each new generation of microbes, like the traits for eye or hair color in our own children, are determined by the genetic material of each organism. This genetic material is dynamic, responding to the environment in ways that sometimes seem mysterious indeed. When there's a threat to the microbe's existence, it can record that threat and through its genetic material alter the constitution of a new generation of microbes, giving the newcomers resistance to materials that might have killed members of their species prior to that.

Modern science has probably caused more rapid and far-reaching changes in the gene pools of the microbial world than any other environmental factor in the history of this planet. Antibiotics and vaccination head the list of innovations that might have nudged the evolutionary processes of microbes, even as we reaped the more obvious benefits of these medical discoveries.

When antibiotics came into widespread use in the 1950s, they were prescribed for everything imaginable, from venereal disease to the common cold. Although we have, in medicine, begun to exercise increasing caution in the use of these drugs, doctors even now give them for acne, for which they are seldom effective. And in many countries to which American manufacturers sell these drugs antibiotics are as available to the general public as cold pills. The only limit placed on their use is the ability to pay for them.

The more these drugs are used, especially at the lower doses, the more they become familiar to the bacterial world. As that knowledge spreads through the microbial world the microbes work overtime to develop their immunities against these drugs. There is plenty of evidence to indicate that this is in fact the case—species that cause human disease are learning to protect themselves against antibiotics. Epidemiologists cite this as one reason for the current epidemics of venereal disease. And it is a major reason that gram-negative infections have become such a problem to patients in hospitals.

Antibiotic resistance occurs in two basic ways in the bacterial world: The first is through the mechanism of evolution that Darwin called *natural selection*. Darwin showed that even in a generation not previously exposed to a particular environmental threat there would be one or more individuals who, unlike their brothers and sisters, would have the capacity for living with that threat. As the less well-adapted members of that generation die out, the well-adapted version of that species multiplies and becomes dominant, carrying to new generations its knowledge of survival. This is as true of the microbial world as it is of the more complex animal world.

A second way that resistance to antibiotics is learned by the bacterial world is through transference of genetic material from one microbe to another. In 1959 Japanese bacteriologists showed that a resistant bacterium is capable of donating a plasmid, that is, genetic knowledge, to a previously vulnerable bacterium simply by briefly touching it. Thus a single resitant bacterium can teach a whole colony of nonresistant bacteria how to defend themselves.

The indiscriminate use of antibiotics ultimately poses a real threat to the doctor within. On the most obvious level it means that at those rare times in life when we need the help of an antibiotic to aid our doctor within, that aid may not be available. The misuse of antibiotics has caused the microbe to evolve a powerful resistance not only to the drug but to the best efforts of our natural healing systems.

USING ANTIBIOTICS EFFECTIVELY

There are certainly times in life when antibiotics can mean the difference between life and death, or between a long recuperation period and a short one. The question arises, how can you make use of these drugs in a way that is helpful rather than harmful to your doctor within? It can be done if you follow these simple but important rules:

1. Remember that antibiotics work *only* on bacteria. They have no effect on viruses. Before you accept an antibiotic prescription from your doctor, discuss this matter with him. Make sure he is certain that what you have is a bacterial infection and, if so, that your immunity system will not be able to deal with it unaided. If your doctor knows that you want to minimize the use of antibiotics, he or she will probably be even more likely to prescribe them only in times of extreme need.

2. Too often people take an antibiotic until their symptoms go away and then they discontinue the drug. At this point the bacteria have usually not all been knocked out. With the antibiotic attack momentarily subsiding, the microbes can now regroup, exchange genetic information about how to resist that drug, and be ready with their own resistance when or if that attack comes again. The full course of an antibiotic treatment includes enough of the drug to prevent this regrouping and exchange of microbial information.

When you do have a bacterial infection that both you and

your physician have decided should be treated with antibiotics, make certain you get an antibiotic that will be powerful enough to knock it out quickly and completely. Always take *all* the antibiotics a doctor prescribes. The only time to discontinue use is if you manifest an allergic reaction. If you have a rash, the most common allergic reaction, or any other suspicious response, discontinue your use of the drug and get in touch with your doctor immediately.

3. Antibiotic treatment can also disrupt the bacterial ecosystems of your digestive tract. The normal production of vitamin K and the B vitamins can thus be impaired. This, of course, is one reason why antibiotics should be taken only with great discretion. During such times you can help your doctor within by making certain you take in foods that are rich in the B vitamins, that is, protein foods and whole cereals. In addition, many physicians now recommend that patients on antibiotics eat large amounts of a good quality, fresh, acidophilus yogurt, since it contains bacteria that encourage the growth of vitamin K in your intestines.

PROTECTING BACTERIAL ECOSYSTEMS FROM HOUSEHOLD CLEANING AND PERSONAL HYGIENE PRODUCTS

There is a mantle made up of dead cells, natural oils, and selected bacteria on the outermost layer of our skin. This mantle, which is necessary to our health and well-being, can be destroyed by chemicals such as household cleaning preparations, even dishwashing detergent. The most obvious example of damage like this is "detergent burn," or dishpan hands, where continuous immersion in strong detergents strips the mantle from the skin. With the protective mantle removed the skin is open to infection, or it simply becomes cracked and raw.

Happily, there are alternatives available to us through which we can take action, on a daily basis, to protect our bacterial ecosystems from destruction by cleansers and other household and personal hygiene products.

Using milder detergents or wearing rubber gloves when using household cleansers can protect your skin from damage. It is a simple way to cooperate with your doctor within, although it may be a minor inconvenience to you.

Similarly, minor skin problems such as dry skin, oily skin, and dandruff may be caused by chemicals in soaps and shampoos, even soaps and shampoos advertised as helping to correct these problems.

In recent years a small number of manufacturers have begun to make personal hygiene products that are "pH balanced." This means that the product will not destroy the normal mantle of your skin, nor will it destroy the protective oils on your hair and scalp. The acidity of the soap or shampoo is matched to the acidity of your skin.

The origin of so many unnecessary health problems seems to be our fear of odors. In this regard, the feminine douche, now available in prepackaged form, is one of the personal hygiene products that produces the greatest problems for our doctor within. For many years it has been known by the medical community that douching upsets the normal microbial balance of a person's vagina. As a result of douching, women can suffer everything from irritated mucosal tissue to vaginitis.

Sore underarms and rashes in the underarm can almost always be traced to the use of deodorants or antiperspirants. Underarm rashes can be caused by allergic reactions to chemicals in your antiperspirant or deodorant, or by irritation that can result when normal bacteria in an area are destroyed, thus allowing foreign invaders that destroy tissue to set up household there.

Antiperspirants are chemicals that inhibit the normal actions of sweat glands; that is, they prevent you from sweating. Deodorants without antiperspirants simply cover up the odor. Of the two, deodorants without antiperspirants have the least damaging effect on your body.

Bear in mind that even though you use an antiperspirant, your body's need to sweat continues. In hot weather, a person doing hard physical labor can sweat from one and one-half to three and three-quarter quarts per hour! Of course, not all of this comes through the underarms, but your underarms are very richly endowed with sweat glands and to inhibit them definitely taxes other areas. You may find, for example, that the use of an underarm antiperspirant causes an increase in the temperature and moisture of your genital area, an area which, like your underarms, is richly endowed with sweat glands. Or you may find that your back or brows sweat more.

Deodorants and antiperspirants may not be at all necessary in solving perspiration odor problems. In recent years, medical researchers have begun investigating the postulate that zinc supplements in the diet can eliminate perspiration odor, regardless of how much a person sweats. Combinations of zinc and vitamin B_6 have also been found useful.* Remember, both zinc and vitamin B_6 are micronutrients that are necessary to health. Neither of them is a drug. How much should you take? In the book *The Practical Encyclopedia of Natural Healing,*† the authors state that thirty milligrams of zinc per day *has* been reported to stop body odor. Take your B_6 in a B-complex formula or multivitamin and mineral formula. Two milligrams of vitamin B_6 is the recommended daily requirement, but under stress a person may use much more than that.

A more conservative remedy for odors will seem obvious, but remember, long before the invention of hygiene sprays and roll-ons, we were able to live together, seeming to get along. Washing your underarms more frequently may be all the protection you need.

FURTHER READING

Bennett, Hal Z. *Cold Comfort*. New York: Clarkson N. Potter, 1979.

Dixon, Bernard. *Magnificent Microbes*. New York: Atheneum, 1979.

Ferguson, Tom, ed. *Medical Self-Care*. New York: Summit Books, 1980.

Glasser, Ronald J. *The Body Is the Hero*. New York: Bantam Books, 1979.

Thomas, Lewis. *The Lives of a Cell*. New York: Bantam Books, 1975.

Travis, John. *Wellness Workbook*. Wellness Associates, 42 Miller Avenue, Mill Valley, Ca. 94941. 1979.

---

* Mark Bricklin, ed., *The Practical Encylopedia of Natural Healing* (Emmaus, Pa.: Rodale Press, Inc., 1976).
† Ibid.

2.

High-Technology Weapons to Fight Disease

IT IS OBVIOUS, with blood being pumped through the human body at the rate of sixty quarts per hour, that once a microbe enters the system it can spread rapidly, infecting many areas of the body at once. The doctor within has to work quickly and efficiently to detect, let's say, a bacterium that has entered through a cut in the finger, before it gets into the bloodstream and is carried off to the brain, or heart, or some other vital organ.

In most diseases that cause serious enough symptoms to make you take notice, there is some fever and/or inflammation involved. These, in fact, are so common that we would be quite justified in labeling them the *universal symptoms* of disease. Usually, these symptoms are not symptoms of disease so much as symptoms of healing. They are events created by your doctor within in response to the presence of disease. The fact that these responses are built into your body, that they are initiated from the inside rather than from the outside, suggests that they are tools of your doctor within.

Within the hypothalamus gland, located in your brain, is a

mechanism that acts like a thermostat. This thermostat is normally set at a temperature between 97°F and 99°F (most of us have been taught that 98.6°F is normal, but the range is actually more broad). When bacteria or viruses are present, your body produces *pyrogens*—a loose translation from the Greek roots meaning "fire starters." The pyrogens signal the hypothalamus to set your thermostat at a higher temperature. This done, hormones from the hypothalamus cause your metabolic rates to increase, thus producing more heat at the same time that blood vessels to skin surfaces are constricted, reducing heat loss from those surfaces. Naturally, as you produce more heat inside you, and that heat is held inside, your overall body temperature rises.

Fever within the range from 99°F to 105°F can be considered a normal response to infection and can usually be reduced by aspirin or other antipyretic medication (literally translated, *antipyretic* means "against or opposed to fire"), or by cold showers or baths. If your body temperature rises above 105°F or falls below 95°F, your doctor within may need outside medical assistance.

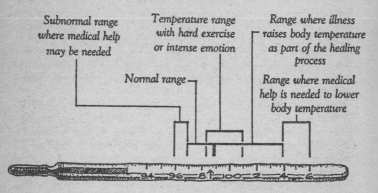

Subnormal range where medical help may be needed

Temperature range with hard exercise or intense emotion

Range where illness raises body temperature as part of the healing process

Normal range

Range where medical help is needed to lower body temperature

Although there has been little or no research done to support the theory that fever does aid in healing, we have a number of indications that this is so. Because viruses have been shown to thrive in temperatures slightly below normal body temperature, it stands to reason that the increased body temperature of fever would reduce viral populations. The higher temperatures are accompanied by higher metabolic rates, which means that everything in the body, including the healing process, has been accelerated. The increase in heart rate brings an increase in the quantities of the healing substances carried by the blood to the infected area. Increases in heart rate also increase the flow of lymph (more about lymph in chapter 3). With these activities speeded up, it is obvious that healing is enhanced.

Inflammation, too, is a healing response without which even a mild infection could become fatal. The fact that it is implicated in the pain of breaks and sprains, arthritis, sinus infections, earaches, colds, flu, and other maladies explains why most of us think of inflammation as an enemy.

Whenever there is tissue damage as a result of disease or injury, the damaged tissue cells produce *histamines*. These histamines cause changes in tiny blood vessels, which in turn release fluids into the injured area. Local blood flow increases, bringing blood cells whose specialty is destroying foreign microbes to the area. Along with these disease-preventing cells comes *fibrinogen*, which causes clotting. The clotting results in what doctors call "walling off," that is, your doctor within literally builds a partition between the infected area and the rest of your body. The effect is to prevent the infection from spreading. The partition, or wall, stops body fluids from moving outside the infected area, and these fluids build up in the area, causing the characteristic swelling of inflammation. That's why your ankle puffs up when you sprain it and why your nose gets stuffy when you have a cold. The buildup of fluid presses on local nerve receptors, inducing pain.

In extreme cases, severe inflammation in untreated infectious diseases can choke off affected organs or cause the growth of fibrous tissue that impairs the organs' normal functions. The inflammation produced by an ear infection, if prolonged, can cause the eardrum to rupture and bleed, leaving the area open to extremely serious infections. The inflammation of a sinus infection can cause debilitating discomfort and can become a *pocket* of infection that drains energy from the rest of the body. In those rare cases inflammation can be harmful but most of the time it helps create health.

White Blood Cells: Multipurpose Healing Tools

After the infected area is walled off, the doctor within can concentrate on healing the wound. He sends white blood cells to the area to clean up debris such as pieces of dead tissue and bacteria.

White blood cells come in many forms. There are some that attack and destroy potential disease agents by surrounding and digesting them. There are other white blood cells that form *antibodies*, that is, protein substances programmed to identify and destroy only specific bacteria or viruses. There are still other white blood cells that aid in clotting and healing wounds. All white blood cells are produced and stored in bone marrow and lymph tissue located throughout your body.

The presence of an increased number of white blood cells in your blood indicates that your doctor within has detected a source of disease in your system and has speeded up the production of white blood cells to combat that threat. Because this occurs, physicians use blood counts to diagnose disease. Let's say that fever, lack of energy, or an achy feeling leads you to seek medical help. A blood sample is taken and the number of white blood cells is high. This is a sure sign that infection is occurring.

White blood cells also can neutralize some of the toxins that may be emitted by bacteria in the course of an infection. Similarly, these cells are reading the antigens of the bacteria (see page 34) and are carrying this information to areas in your body where your doctor within is creating antibodies.

Rebuilding Damaged Tissue

Even as all this is taking place in your body, your doctor within is synthesizing protein substances for closing up the original wound, if that was the site of infection, or is rebuilding tissue that has been damaged by disease. (See illustration.) New tissue cells are being born to replace the old ones damaged by the original cut or the infection. And new blood vessels are growing to bring nutrients to the healing tissue.

The capacity of your doctor within to rebuild tissue damaged by physical trauma or infection is truly amazing. Although the mysteries of these regenerative processes rival those of birth itself, there are some parts that are quite accessible to us. Rather than attempt to explain these processes by words alone, I've provided some illustrations on the next page.

Phagocytes: The Mobile Patrol Force of the Doctor Within

Biologists tell us that one of the most sophisticated tools we have for detecting and neutralizing foreign substances may be related to an interesting but primitive microorganism that lives in octopuses. These microorganisms seem to wander about aimlessly in the octopuses, where they make their homes. Whenever they bump into an intruder in that organism, they respond by chewing it up. These primitive microorganisms appear to have lives quite separate from the octopus. It is almost as though they have stumbled in and set up housekeeping by chance.

In the human body, cells very much like the ones I've just described are produced and stored in our bone marrow. Millions of them circulate in our bloodstream. But instead of wandering aimlessly, finding intruders by chance, these cells seem to have developed radar systems to track down intruders the instant they enter our bodies. In human beings these cells are called *phagocytes* (pronounced fag-oh-sights), a word derived from the Greek, meaning "cell eaters." The phagocytes are members of the white blood cell family.

HOW THE DOCTOR WITHIN HEALS A WOUND

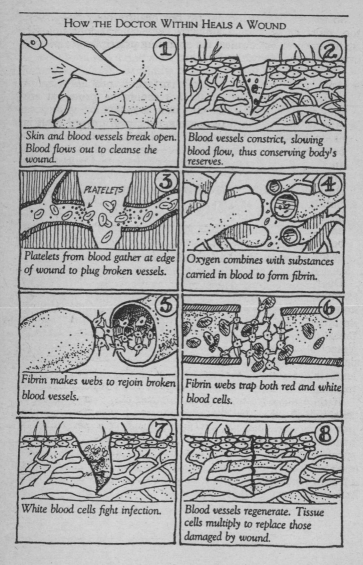

1 Skin and blood vessels break open. Blood flows out to cleanse the wound.

2 Blood vessels constrict, slowing blood flow, thus conserving body's reserves.

3 PLATELETS Platelets from blood gather at edge of wound to plug broken vessels.

4 Oxygen combines with substances carried in blood to form fibrin.

5 Fibrin makes webs to rejoin broken blood vessels.

6 Fibrin webs trap both red and white blood cells.

7 White blood cells fight infection.

8 Blood vessels regenerate. Tissue cells multiply to replace those damaged by wound.

So that these cells do not eat our healthy body cells, they, too, must be able to distinguish between self and not-self. Stated in three basic rules, the operating principles for phagocytes might go something like this:

- Any substance with a rough surface is probably an intruder, since the body cells that should be protected are smooth. Rough-surfaced substances should be chewed up.
- Any substance that exerts a magnetic pull toward itself is likely to be an intruder, too. Most substances within the body have electronegative surface charges and so repel one another. Dead tissue and foreign particles that might enter the body are frequently electropositive and should be chewed up.
- Substances such as the membranes of dead tissue cells also have rough surfaces and electropositive charges. The naturally occurring debris of cells constantly dying and being replaced should be cleaned up, or the normal clutter of life will clog our veins and arteries.

Once it has identified the intruder, the phagocyte becomes extremely excited. Under a microscope you can see it dancing around, seeming to act out an ancient rite as it centers in on its target. The phagocyte finally clutches the intruder to its breast and throws long tentacles around it. For a moment the tentacles look like the tentacles of an octopus clutching a delicious morsel for its supper. But then the phagocyte's tentacles—technically, they're pseudopods—appear to fuse together. The intruder is totally engulfed by the phagocyte.

If the phagocyte has located a bacterium, it may inject it with a deadly chemical. For example, the phagocyte might inject hydrogen peroxide—produced inside the phagocyte—which oxidizes substances the bacterium needs for its own survival. Finally, it secretes enzymes that quickly digest whatever remains of the intruder. Depending on the size and type of phagocyte, it may go on to neutralize up to twenty bacteria until, having fulfilled its purpose in life, it dies.

Antibodies: White Blood Cells That Define the Enemy

Once it enters the human body a bacterium or a virus is its own worst enemy. It can go undetected by the doctor within for only a brief period. Special white blood cells called *antibodies* are formed within your body to match the microbe's surface characteristics and ultimately cause its destruction. Certain areas of each bacterium's surface have tiny protuberances that identify it as a member of one bacteria family or another. These protuberances are called *antigens*.

Each bacterium or virus has its own pattern of antigens, and each will call for a particular pattern of antibodies. Like the characteristics that make dogs recognizable as dogs, cats recognizable as cats, and humans recognizable as humans, the antigens of each family of bacteria characterize members of that group. Some antigens are conical in shape, while others may be shaped like a club or even a series of rectangles. The shape, size, and patterns of these characteristics vary widely, but within any family of microbes all will have characteristics that identify them as members of that family.

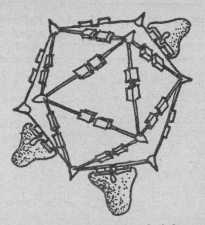

A virus with antibodies (represented by shaded areas) attaching themselves to antigens

In the illustration, notice the shaded configurations that look like puzzle pieces being pressed into place on the antigen sites. These represent antibodies, created by the doctor within, fitted into place on the bacterium and already marking it for destruction.

When a bacterium enters your system your doctor within somehow manages to identify that intruder by "reading" its antigens. Some scientists believe that certain white blood cells read the antigen patterns and carry that information to lymph nodes, where antibodies are created. Others believe that phagocytes destroy the intruders and carry pieces of them, with their antigens still in place, to the lymph nodes, where they are analyzed by the doctor within. There is good reason to believe that both these mechanisms work together in the body.

Somehow—the process is not fully understood by scientists—the doctor within creates antibodies to clip on to the antigens. These antibodies flow out into every area of your body, clipping on to only those surfaces that have antigens to match them. One way antibodies do their work is by interrupting the metabolic processes of bacteria. When antibodies attach themselves to the antigens of a bacterium they interfere with its feeding mechanisms. The bacterium, in this way deprived of nutrients, literally starves to death.

Through antibodies, the doctor within is able to "tag" notself substances with extreme accuracy. Because each microbe is so specifically coded, there is little room for error and little danger that an antibody will attach to a healthy tissue cell. This biological fail-safe system gives the doctor within tremendous power to locate and destroy an infinite variety of not-self substances while posing no threat to healthy tissue.

As though to provide an extra margin of safety for the self, the doctor within adds still another step to the process. The antibodies do not themselves neutralize or destroy the microbe. Instead, they attract something called *complement*, a substance made by your doctor within. The complement targets in on the surface of a microbe that has been tagged with antibodies, somehow attracted to the area by the antigen-antibody link.

There are nine complements, and these arrange themselves on the surface of the microbe in a doughnut-shaped configuration. (See illustration below.) The center of the doughnut forms a pore, and this pore grows into a hole on the surface of the microbe. What follows is a little like the popping of a balloon, which is, of course, fatal to the microbe. Phagocytes, which have no trouble whatsoever identifying particles of the broken microbe as not-self, now come in and clean up the area. The phagocyte may then carry harmless pieces of the microbe, which still contains antigens, back to lymph nodes, where the further production of antibodies is stimulated. This whole process takes time, but once the doctor within has identified the surface configurations of a microbe, he logs this information into a memory bank. That memory bank is what makes long-term immunity and protection by vaccination possible.

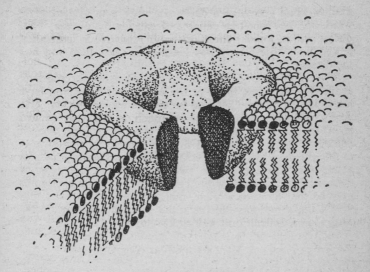

Complement forms a doughnut-shaped hole on the surface of the microbe, leading to its destruction.

THE SEVEN-DAY CURE: FROM BACTERIA TO THE LASTING PROTECTION OF ANTIBODIES

Your doctor within doesn't create specialized antibodies to neutralize new microbes instantly. For most microbes, a week or ten days is needed between the time that a bacterium or virus first enters your system and the time your doctor within has created enough antibodies to neutralize it. That, basically, is why most infectious diseases last from a week to ten days—not because the disease *wears itself out* but because it takes that long for your doctor within to create the antibodies.

In most cases, however, the week or so necessary for creating a set of antibodies is required only once in a lifetime. After the doctor within has figured out the disease and has stored that information in his memory bank, you won't be bothered by that disease again. The microbes that caused mumps when you were a child can enter your system afterward, but they won't be capable of causing the disease. Your doctor within knocks them out with ready-made antibodies, antibodies whose recipe was learned the first time you had the disease.

Why, if this is true, do we get some diseases over and over again? For example, think of the number of times you have had colds or the flu. Cold and flu viruses evolve quickly. This year's cold virus can change so much in the year or two ahead that your doctor within won't even recognize it when it comes up again. It will seem to be a completely new virus—as, indeed, it is. In addition, it is known that there are at least a hundred different viruses that cause colds, and each of these is constantly evolving. Though the physical symptoms may be the same, or similar, the antigens on the virus that causes the symptoms can be quite different. So the doctor within has a difficult time indeed keeping up.

VACCINATION: A MEANS OF EDUCATING THE DOCTOR WITHIN

Certain advances in medical science have provided us with tools that aid your doctor within in building antibodies against disease. A few infections to which the human race is prone truly tax the doctor within to the limit. Polio, tetanus, and rabies are excellent examples. Ideally, your immune system will form antibodies to even these diseases, but this takes time, and time can be of the essence. Can your doctor within neutralize the not-self substances before they cause permanent damage or even death? This race for health is, happily, an issue in only a relatively small number of common infectious diseases.

Back in the late 1700s, a doctor by the name of Edward Jenner observed that people who worked around cows in English rural districts never got smallpox. He observed that the people with immunity did, however, report having once had a disease called "cowpox," with mild physical symptoms that resembled smallpox. He hypothesized that it was the cowpox that somehow provided these people with smallpox immunity.

Jenner devised a daring experiment. Making scratches on the arms of people who'd never had smallpox, he smeared the scratches with pus taken from the lesions of people with cowpox. No one in this test group suffered any physical symptoms of cowpox, except for a small amount of festering around the vaccination wound. Jenner continued to observe these people for years and discovered that none of them ever contracted smallpox, the more serious disease, even though they were living in the midst of smallpox epidemics. He not only proved that vaccination could work but that one disease could sometimes provide immunity from another. (We now know that this occurs because of the similarities in antigen patterns on the surfaces of certain different families of bacteria or viruses.)

The experiments of Edward Jenner provided important evidence for the existence of a mysterious inner system for neutralizing disease-causing substances that might enter our bodies. Once the human body had learned to neutralize disease-causing substances, that knowledge seemed to stay with it for years, often for a lifetime. Jenner's experiments revolutionized medicine and led to what is now almost total universal freedom from smallpox, a disease that once ravaged thousands of people.

Vaccination has been much refined since Jenner's day but the basic principles are the same. Nowadays, we receive vaccines for a wide range of diseases: smallpox, measles, tetanus, diphtheria, polio, and even the flu. And the vaccines produce no noticeable physical symptoms whatsoever. The reasons for this are twofold: First, dosages of live vaccine can be kept low enough to teach your doctor within how to produce antibodies while causing no apparent disease symptoms; second, it has been discovered that your body can read antigens on the surfaces of microbes that have been killed and that can no longer cause disease. Thus microbe particles that pose no health threat can give your doctor within the raw materials for creating antibodies. These antibodies will protect you from the specific disease the live members of that microbe family might cause.

Vaccination can offer you a way of educating your doctor within while minimizing your own discomfort or fear of contracting the actual disease. The following table provides you with a list of diseases for which vaccines are available.

DISEASES FOR WHICH VACCINES ARE AVAILABLE

NAME OF DISEASE	Comments
CHOLERA	Vaccine available. The disease is most prevalent in Asia, Africa, and the Middle East. Can be prevented through sanitary disposal of human wastes. Vaccine protects for about 6 months.
COMMON COLD	Vaccines available for a limited number of viruses that cause colds, but only those that are offered for potential military epidemics are effective. Vaccines that are offered for public use are not effective.
DIPHTHERIA	Vaccine available. Routine administration to children has stopped the threat of this disease in U.S. It is given as part of DPT (diphtheria/pertussis/tetanus) shots.
MEASLES	Vaccines available. Live vaccines are used and produce mild measles symptoms in about 5% of people vaccinated.
MUMPS	Vaccine available.
PERTUSSIS (WHOOPING COUGH)	Vaccine available. It is given as part of DPT shots.
PLAGUE—PESTIS (BUBONIC PLAGUE)	Vaccines available. These bacteria are carried by rodents and fleas infesting them. Disease is now rare, thanks to modern control of rodents in cities.
POLIO	Vaccines available. Salk vaccine, by shots, has been replaced by Sabin vaccine, given orally. Sabin is more effective. Disease has been nearly annihilated by vaccine programs.
RABIES	Vaccination of domestic animals minimizes danger to humans. After being bitten by a rabid animal, humans can

get vaccination treatment to prevent rabies. Vaccines are also available for people working in professions where animal bites are common.

RUBELLA (GERMAN OR THREE-DAY MEASLES)	Vaccine available. Given mainly to prevent congenital problems of unborn children. Should never be given during pregnancy.
SMALLPOX	Vaccine available. No longer routinely given to children. Vaccination mainly important when traveling to other countries where smallpox is common.
TETANUS	Vaccine available. It is given as part of DPT shot. Boosters are recommended every ten years. With deep cuts, booster should be given if patient hasn't had one in three years.
TUBERCULOSIS	Vaccine available. Since TB is now rare, vaccine is used mostly to protect people in intimate contact with someone infected with TB. Also used in treatment programs.
TYPHOID FEVER	Vaccine available. Given only to people actually exposed.
YELLOW FEVER	Vaccines available. Given only at Public Health Service Yellow Fever Vaccination Centers in the U.S. when outbreak is indicated or when a person will be living in high-incidence area. Mosquito control is the main protection against this disease.

Killer Cells: Cloak-and-Dagger Agents for the Doctor Within

A virus, unlike most bacteria, has no supporting structures of its own—its exists entirely inside cells. It cannot absorb or digest food, nor can it metabolize nutrients to produce energy. It is like a brain without a body. It is, except for the protein sheath that surrounds it, pure genetic material.

Viruses infect us by entering our tissue cells and using them to reproduce more of their own. Once inside our cells, viruses escape detection by the antibodies, which are looking for antigens with which to hook up. Because there are no antigens on tissue cells, the antibodies find nothing out of the ordinary and so do nothing, which is exactly what they are programmed to do.

Killer cells, on the other hand, are able to detect activity going on inside our cells. Scientists don't fully understand how this is done but one theory is that they feel the surfaces of infected cells. A cell infected with a virus becomes distorted and wrinkled. Although an antibody won't respond to this surface, the killer cell will. The latter attaches itself to the infected cell and injects chemical compounds that evolved hundreds of millions of years ago into the cytoplasm of that cell. Like poisonous gases, these chemicals completely annihilate every virus that might be hiding there. The work of the killer cell is fast, direct, and thorough.

Killer cells are born in the lymph nodes and begin their lives as lymphocytes (which we will discuss in the next chapter). They go after potential disease-causing agents with the single-mindedness of kamikaze pilots, homing in on their targets as though guided by radio control, and, once locked in on their targets, killer cells are truly ruthless.

Killer cells are important tools in preventing or healing viral infections ranging from the flu to encephalitis and Rocky Mountain spotted fever. Research indicates that certain forms of cancer may be caused by viruses, too, viruses that can be controlled by the tools of your doctor within.

KILLER CELLS AND CANCER

It is now believed that most cancer cells are nothing more than our own body cells gone haywire; for one of a dozen or more reasons, a new cell may contain genetic material that is altered. Scientists speculate that genetic material is altered in one of three possible ways: by chemicals, by radiation, and by viruses that enter healthy cells and transform them into cancer cells. These cancer cells, along with their progeny, don't know what to do—except reproduce. These cells are not "coded" to become useful cells in a muscle, liver, lung, or any part of the body. Instead, they reproduce willy-nilly, and, with nowhere to go and nothing to do, their useless colonies eventually crowd out healthy and productive tissue.

Most medical researchers now commonly believe that cancer cells are always being produced in our bodies. They usually die out of their own accord, like the ill-fated dinosaurs of old. But those that do survive elude the weapon we have in antibodies; they are less successful at eluding killer cells.

Because cancer cells have many of the same attributes as normal tissue cells and even use the same blood supplies, they fail to provoke the antibody system to act. It stands to reason that antibodies, which are designed to leave healthy cells alone, would also ignore cancer cells that resemble healthy cells. The killer cell, however, does an excellent job of locating and destroying these abnormal cells—again, by feeling the wrinkles or other abnormal characteristics on the surface of the cancer cell. On a daily basis the doctor within patrols your entire body, ready with killer cells to knock out any cancer cells that might survive. Ordinarily this is done with ease.

You may ask why the doctor within sometimes fails to clean up defective cells, thus allowing tumors to grow. The answer is complex. Some cancer cells, for example, cause the creation of *immunosuppressants*, substances that reduce the power of the immunity system. And sometimes, as the result of being subjected to radiation or chemical contamination (through industrial pollution, smoking, or the ingestion of chemicals in our food) a large amount of damage occurs to genetic material. When the damage is too widespread, the doctor within can't keep up with the demand. It isn't that the doctor within fails to do his job, it is that the person with the tumor has, for one reason or another, become subjected to more contaminants than the tools of the doctor within were designed to handle.

Interferon: Birth Control for the Viruses That Threaten You

Another important tool of the doctor within is interferon, a protein substance produced inside tissue cells. Like killer cells, interferon has the power to detect and combat viruses, sometimes in conjunction with killer cells and sometimes alone.

The presence of a virus in a cell touches off a series of chemical events that results in the production of interferon, which is poisonous to the virus but harmless to the cells. Rather than killing the virus, as chemical compounds from killer cells do, interferon "interferes" with the virus's reproduction. In most cases it doesn't completely stop reproduction; it simply slows it down.

Scientists are only beginning to understand interferon. They know that each of our cells appears to have the ability to produce it. But production doesn't start until at least a few cells are destroyed by viral infection. The process goes something like this: A single virus enters a cell and begins reproducing inside the cell. The newborn viruses escape, going out to infect still other cells. The original infected cell slowly dies, but before it does it releases interferon into the fluids that surround it. Interferon produced by the dying cell is then taken up by healthy cells, which begin producing it on their own. As the production of interferon increases, the viruses are literally driven off; they are unable to enter the cells, where they can reproduce. Interferon acts like a birth-control program, prohibiting the virus from making more of its kind.

Though the presence of a virus is probably the primary signal for the production of interferon, it has been found that body temperatures above 103°F can also initiate the process. Research cited by Linus Pauling has shown that large quantities of vitamin C may also encourage tissue cells in interferon production. Stress has been found to have an opposite effect. Even when the circumstances that would otherwise cause interferon to be produced—i.e., the presence of a virus—are clearly there, in times of stress the production of interferon is reduced.

Most healing tools for infectious disease originate outside the infected tissue, either starting their lives in lymph or in the special blood cells in the bloodstream. Interferon, however, originates inside infected cells, doing its work in the cytoplasm of the cell itself rather than in the blood, lymph, or interstitial fluids, as antibodies and killer cells do.

In some ways, interferon works on viruses on the same principle as our man-made antibiotics work on bacteria. It interrupts viral reproduction, or kills viruses directly, through toxins that are fatal to the virus and harmless to the tissue cell. While bacteria live and reproduce outside our cells, viruses live and reproduce inside our cells, where man-made antibiotics can have no effect on them. In this respect interferon and antibiotics differ: Interferon works on viruses, not bacteria.

In recent years medical science has been attempting to synthesize chemical equivalents of interferon, or to make medicines available that will stimulate our cells to produce it. Some scientists look upon this work as the next big breakthrough in medicine's struggle to gain power over infectious disease. If the equivalent of interferon, or an inducer, is ever reproduced by the chemists, and I believe it will be, we will then have a medication as effective against viral infection as antibiotics now are against bacterial infection.

INTERFERON AS A POTENTIAL CURE FOR CANCER

Up until now, medical researchers were pessimistic about ever being able to develop a drug that would work inside our cells, making life unbearable for viruses while leaving healthy tissue alone. Injections of interferon may change all that.

Recently the American Cancer Society has funded one of the most generous research grants of its history to test the effects of interferon injections on cancer patients. Many types of cancer are known to be caused by viruses, and so it stands to reason that interferon, like killer cells, holds much promise for combating this disease.

Unlike other forms of antiviral therapies, including radiation and chemotherapy using drugs such as amantadine and methisazone, interferon appears to create no health hazards of its own. Side effects, if any, are negligible. The reason, of course, is that the human body itself produces interferon. This healing substance is fully compatible with healthy tissue, and fully effective against most viruses.

Why, you may ask, if the body normally produces this substance, would it become necessary to inject more of it from the outside to heal a disease such as cancer? The answer is not simple, but it boils down to this single issue: Under certain circumstances viruses are able to reproduce themselves quicker than your body can reproduce sufficient quantities of interferon. By learning to produce interferon in larger quantities, we're able to reduce viral populations to levels your doctor within can comfortably handle.

The early results are promising. In fact, they are so promising that pharmaceutical companies in this country alone have poured $150 million into research and production facilities.* And the National Cancer Institute has put in an order for up to $9 million worth of interferon for further studies.

At present, production of interferon is extremely expensive and its application is limited to life-threatening disease. The average interferon treatment for a cancer victim costs about $150 per day, with the price tag for a complete course of treatment at about $30,000. However, new techniques for producing interferon will soon reduce its cost to about 5 percent of these figures. In the future, it is conceivable that as the price of interferon treatment goes down it will be available for any number of diseases caused by viruses. Some limited research has already been done demonstrating its effectiveness in the treatment of hepatitis.

---

* "Interferon: The IF Drug for Cancer," *Time*, March 31, 1980.

FURTHER READING

Galton, Lawrence. *Medical Advances.* New York: Penguin Books, 1979.

Guyton, Arthur C. *Textbook of Medical Physiology,* 5th ed. Philadelphia: W. B. Saunders Company, 1976.

The Harvard Medical School Health Letter, monthly publication, $15 per year, The Harvard Medical School Health Letter, 79 Garden Street, Cambridge, Mass. 02138.

Kapit, Wynn, and Elson, Lawrence M. *The Anatomy Coloring Book.* New York: Harper & Row, 1977.

Notkins, Abner L., ed. *Viral Immunology and Immunopathology.* New York: Academic Press, 1975.

Sehnert, Keith W., and Eisenberg, Harold. *How to Be Your Own Doctor—Sometimes.* New York: Grosset & Dunlap, 1976.

3.

The Incredible Lymph System: Communication Network of the Doctor Within

THERE IS A MASTER CONTROL SYSTEM through which your doctor within directs most of the workings of his collection of tools for preventing and healing infectious disease. Actually, a second circulatory system, the lymph system, circulates lymph fluid that carries white blood cells called *lymphocytes* throughout your body. These lymphocytes, which start life in your lymph nodes, your spleen, your bones, and other areas of your body, fulfill two important roles: First, they detect and identify not-self substances such as bacteria that cause disease; second, they carry the information they've collected about these substances to areas of your body where cells to neutralize microbial invaders are synthesized. In essence, the lymph system is the communication network for the processes of immunity we discussed earlier.

Imagine, if you will, millions of lymphocytes, with both detection and message-carrying capacities, circulating freely throughout your body. There is hardly a cell they don't explore in great detail in the course of a day.

Whereas the circulation of blood is accomplished mainly by the centrally located pump we call the heart, lymph is pumped through your body by a sort of massage action within the lymph vessels. The squeezing action of the lymph vessels serves as a pump mechanism throughout the body. Although the lymph vessels don't, technically speaking, have muscles like those found in your blood vessels, they do have a fibrous structure that accomplishes pretty much the same thing.

Lymph moves slowly through its vessels. When you're at rest it moves at the rate of about four fluid ounces per hour. There has been little research published on how much lymph is moved during vigorous exercise, but it is known that exercise greatly increases the flow of lymph, just as it increases the flow of blood in your body. One estimate is that lymph may move as much as fifteen times faster during exercise than during rest, which would boost flow from four to sixty ounces an hour. That's a considerable difference in circulating volume!

The reason for an increased rate of lymph circulation during exercise is that the actions of large muscles, around which the lymph vessels flow, massage the walls of these vessels as they contract and relax. The rhythmic motions of the muscles press the vessels and force the fluid to move, just as pressing the sides of a tube of toothpaste causes the contents of the tube to ooze out. Throughout the lymph vessels there are tissue structures that act like one-way valves, keeping the lymph moving in one direction at all times.

Lymphocytes: Microscopic Space Probes

The Greeks and Romans, nearly twenty-four hundred years ago, were the first to study lymph. And, strange as it may seem, most of the theories that prevailed in ancient Greece were still held to be true until only the past few years. The Greeks believed, for example, that lymph nodes, located at various strategic places throughout our bodies, were filters for lymph. They believed that during an infection these nodes trapped microbes picked up by the lymph fluid itself.

The basis for this theory was the observation that the nodes often enlarge when there's an infection present, leading physicians to conclude that microbial material being filtered by the nodes was causing them to swell up in size. The Greek

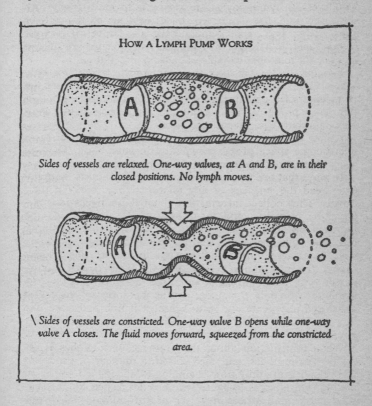

HOW A LYMPH PUMP WORKS

Sides of vessels are relaxed. One-way valves, at A and B, are in their closed positions. No lymph moves.

Sides of vessels are constricted. One-way valve B opens while one-way valve A closes. The fluid moves forward, squeezed from the constricted area.

theory that nodes are simple filters conjures up images of something like oil filters in automobiles, catching and holding the junk that might enter the system. In the past few years, however, this vision has been expanded and corrected. The nodes are not, after all, the simple filters the Greeks thought they were.

What happens is this: Lymphocytes travel throughout the body, eventually channeled through the nodes by a complex network of lymph vessels. In addition to traveling through lymph vessels, a vast network of tubes as complex as the blood vessels, lymphocytes are also able to move freely into the tissue fluid, the uncharted spaces between all the cells of your body. The same lymphocytes also travel into your bloodstream. Wherever they go, the lymphocytes are on the lookout for microbes capable of causing infection.

Imagine, if you will, that each lymphocyte is a microscopic space probe. Aboard each probe is a highly sophisticated set of receptors for examining every surface it contacts. In addition, each probe carries a computer for storing highly complex data that these receptors collect.

At any given time your doctor within has millions of these microscopic space probes circulating in your body. They go everywhere, orbiting every cell, every particle of you.

In ways that are not fully understood by scientists, lymphocytes read the surfaces of any microbes they touch in their travels. They collect information about the antigens identifying these microbes, and they carry what they learn to the lymph nodes. Inside each node a number of important things are done with these data, and as activity increases, the node tends to enlarge. First, what appears to be a sorting process occurs; the information collected by the lymphocytes is compared with other information about antigens that is permanently stored in the node, just as memories of your past are stored in your brain. In this respect lymph nodes are like tiny specialized brains located in hundreds of areas all over your body.

When information about the presence of microbes is received by the nodes, and then sorted, a number of processes that scientists are only now beginning to understand are set in motion. The effect is to cause lymphocytes to become messengers, carrying a whole new set of information into your bloodstream. This information is given to plasma cells and tells them how to produce antibodies specifically programmed to destroy the microbe in question. The plasma cells eventually release antibodies into the bloodstream, and these flood into the areas where the potentially disease-causing microbes temporarily reside.

Compared to your blood system, your lymph system may seem like a sluggish affair. But with the lymph, that slowness may well be an asset. To accomplish all they must, lymphocytes need time, and that time is provided in the slower pace of the lymph system.

Lymph and Exercise

It is ironic that many of the best tools of the doctor within work least well during prolonged periods of reduced physical activity. I say this is ironic because the reflex for most people, when they aren't feeling well, is to lie down and rest, to stop all physical activity. While sleep offers its own healing benefits, there are limits to how much rest is good for you during, let's say, an infection or when you are trying to avoid the latest cold or flu that's going around.

Because of the nature of the lymph system, specifically the pumping actions that take place all along it, physical exercise has a dramatic effect on your doctor within's power to prevent or heal an infection. The benefits of physical exercise will be examined in more detail in chapter 7, but for the purposes of this discussion it is important to keep in mind that exercise stimulates the muscles to contract and relax. The action of the muscles as they press against the lymph vessels moves lymph fluid through your body. In addition to this, movement of your arms and legs, even movement that requires very little physical exertion, causes the lymphatic vessels themselves to stretch and relax, encouraging an increased movement of your lymph fluid.

Probably the subtlest mechanism by which physical activity influences the movements of lymph is arterial pulsation. In many areas of your body lymph vessels closely parallel and even touch your blood vessels. During vigorous exercise, which is twelve minutes or more of aerobic-type activity, the arteries pulsate in strong rhythms, pressing against lymph vessels. This, of course, has the same effect on moving your lymph as pressing the tube has on your toothpaste—though, of course, on a much subtler level.

POSTURES TO GET THE LYMPH MOVING

In yoga you place your body in positions that increase circulation of blood and lymph to areas of your body that might not otherwise get the full attention of these fluids in the course of a regular day. Stop to consider the effect of gravity on your system and the yogi's shoulder stand begins to make sense. All the fluids that normally have to go up can, for a few moments each day, go down.

We know that lymph pumps are stimulated by nearly any change of position. It is interesting to note, however, that most yoga postures achieve at least three of the benefits that improve lymph circulation: (1) stimulation of lymph by the massage-action of muscles and arteries pressing against lymph vessels; (2) movement of limbs and organs into positions that maximize the flow of lymph either because the vessel is momentarily straight instead of turning a corner, or because it can momentarily go down rather than up; (3) increased flexibility of muscles, as well as blood and lymph vessels, through gentle stretching.

The following set of postures, which I call "The Ten," are easy to do and, unlike many of the more advanced yoga postures, they require no special instruction. (However, if you are being treated for muscular or skeletal problems, be sure to consult your physician before doing yoga exercises.) Do The Ten as a set, in sequence. Go easy on yourself as you do them; don't strain. The idea is to make your muscles and lymph system more flexible and to increase circulation. A calm mind and a relaxed body are the real goals of these postures.

Understand that unless you are experienced in yoga or other body techniques The Ten may not be comfortable the first few times you try them, any more than riding a bike for the first few times is comfortable. But over a period of time each posture will get easier and you'll finish up feeling refreshed, relaxed, and renewed.

Establish a quiet time of day to do The Ten. Early in the morning, before breakfast, is ideal. In the evening, at least an hour after eating a light supper, may also be a good time for the postures. At any rate, look for twenty or thirty minutes when you will definitely not be disturbed.

Do the postures in loose-fitting clothes or in underwear so that your clothes won't restrict your movements. A firm surface, such as a padded rug or a thin exercise mat, is recommended.

THE TEN

1. Supine Position: *Lie flat on your back, both heels on the floor, hands by your sides, palms up. Take several deep but easy breaths and let each one out slowly. Use meditation techniques described in chapter 4 to achieve a deeply relaxed state of mind and body.*

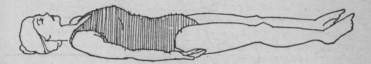

2. Knee Touches: *While still on your back, clasp your hands behind your neck. While keeping your right leg on the floor, lift your left knee toward your chest. Raise your shoulders and turn slightly, touching your right elbow to the inside of your left knee. Do the same on the opposite side. Repeat four to six times for each side.*

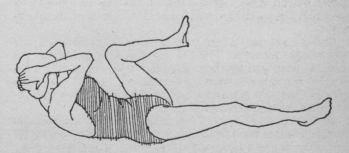

3. Egg Rolls: *Sit up and clasp your hands under your knees. Let your chin relax against your chest. Now raise your knees and rock back on your shoulders. Exhale as you rock back to your buttocks. Rock forward and back and from side to side in fluid, easy movements. Repeat this rocking motion six or eight times.*

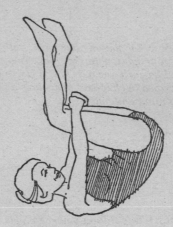

4. Shoulder Stand: *Rock back on your shoulders into a full shoulder stand. Try to get as straight up as you can. Once in this position you'll find you can slowly relax your shoulder muscles, and any discomfort you initially felt will be lessened. Hold this position for whatever length of time is comfortable. That may be only seconds the first time you try it. In time this will extend to five, ten, or even thirty minutes.*

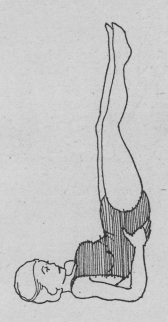

Incidentally, if you have ever had a serious neck injury or if you have a tendency to get a stiff neck, forget about doing shoulder stands. People for whom shoulder stands are not advisable may find they can enjoy pretty much the same benefits on an inclined board, their legs and buttocks placed ten to twelve inches higher than their shoulders.

5. The Cobra: *Lie on your stomach. Relax yourself. Place your hands on the floor as though preparing to do a push-up. Take a deep breath and hold it. Arch your back and rise slowly like a snake, as illustrated. Hold this position until you feel the need for air. Return to your prone position, relax, and exhale slowly. Inhale. Rise slowly again, like a snake. Repeat three times.*

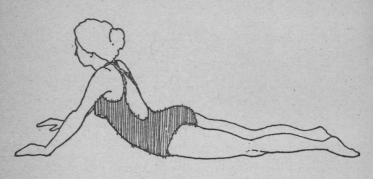

6. Push-up and Bridge: *Lie on your stomach, do a push-up, and raise yourself until your arms are fully extended. Then raise your buttocks so that your body forms an arched bridge. While in this position take several deep breaths, exhale, and then pull in your stomach so that you are drawing your internal organs toward your spine. Hold this position until you feel the need to inhale. Exhale and return to the prone position. Repeat three or four times.*

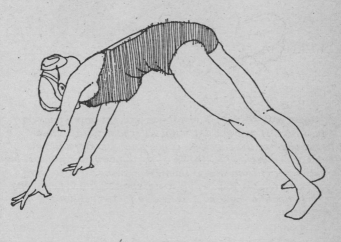

7. Sun Salutations: *Still in a push-up position, let your torso rock back, knees toward your chest, arms extended. Hold this position, stretching your arms and shoulders like a cat in the sun. Breathe easily. Return to a prone position and do it again. Repeat two or three times.*

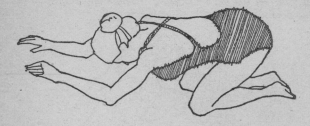

8. Squat and Wiggles: *Squat down and put your hands on your knees. If you find this difficult at first, hold on to a heavy chair or the edge of a couch until you develop your balance and technique. While in the squatting position swing your buttocks from side to side. Then swing them forward and back, tipping your pelvis to accomplish this. Then swing your buttocks around in a circle. Do four repetitions of each movement.*

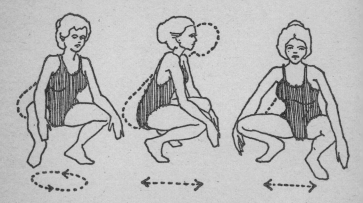

9. Hula Circles: *Place your hands on your hips, feet spread. While keeping your shoulders relatively stationary, swing your hips in a wide circle as though you were spinning a hula hoop. Go clockwise seven or eight turns. Stop. Then go counterclockwise seven or eight turns.*

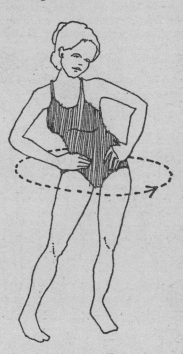

10. Side Bends: *From the Hula Circles starting position, spread your legs so that your feet are approximately three feet apart, toes pointed out. Bend to one side, reaching for your toes, exhaling. Return to a full standing position, then reach toward the toes of the opposite foot. When reaching toward the right, let your right knee bend while keeping your left leg straight. Do the same for the other side. Exhale as you touch your toes. Inhale as you rise. Do six or more repetitions for each side.*

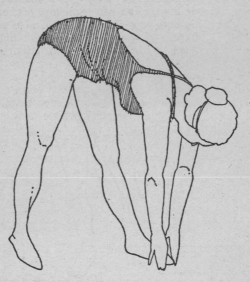

To finish off The Ten run in place for a few minutes, letting your arms and upper torso be very loose. You should feel yourself jangling around like a dancing puppet.

MASSAGE TO STIMULATE THE LYMPH

Daily massage to stimulate your lymph system is probably best done through self-massage unless, of course, you are fortunate enough to have your own live-in masseur or masseuse.

Lie on your back, assuming the Supine Position described

in the beginning of The Ten. Let yourself be relaxed. Use meditation to achieve deep relaxation (meditation techniques will be described in chapter 4). Ideally, do this in the nude.

A GENTLE TOUCH

While in the Supine Position, raise your arms toward the ceiling, being languorous and slow in your movements. Touch the tips of your fingers and rub them together, experiencing the sensations in both your right and left hand as you do this.

Draw the fingers of your left hand with light pressure down the full length of your right arm, continuing all the way to the center of your sternum (breastbone). The massage should be *caressing* rather than *pressing*, so that the caressing arm can stay quite relaxed. (It takes only a small amount of pressure to stimulate the lymph vessels.) Do this three or four times for each arm. Always massage from the most distant point of your body into the center of your sternum, since that will be the direction of the lymph flow you want to stimulate.

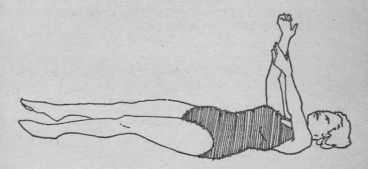

Rest your arms on your chest for a moment and let yourself enjoy the sensations you are feeling.

Place the fingers of both hands on your forehead. Slowly massage your face, drawing your fingers from your forehead down to your chin several times, using the same caressing rather than pressing movements as before.

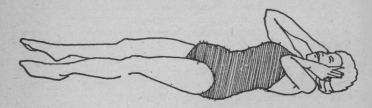

Rest your hands on your chest again. Enjoy the sensations you are feeling on your face.

Rest your arms at your sides, touching the outsides of your thighs as far down as you can reach without stretching. Now draw your fingers up along your thighs, across your belly, up to the center of your sternum. Then do the same from the tops of your thighs to your sternum. Then draw your fingers from your genital area to your sternum.

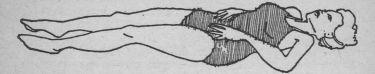

Rest as before and enjoy the sensations you are feeling.

Raise one knee toward your chest and, without straining, massage with both hands from your foot, up along your calf to your knee, down your thigh to your pelvis, up across your belly to the center of your sternum. Do this several times for each leg.

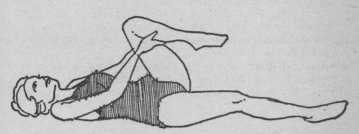

Return to the Supine Position and enjoy the sensations of the leg massage. Then massage both arms, as you did in the beginning.

Let yourself stay relaxed and enjoy the sensations of the massage for several minutes before you get up, realizing as you do that you are aiding your doctor within.

If you have a partner to work with, all the better. Follow essentially the same instructions as you massage your partner or your partner massages you. In addition to the instructions above, you and your partner will be able to massage your backs. When massaging the back, follow the same principles as you did in the self-massage, that is, go from the outer extremities *toward* the center of your sternum—or the center of the back, in this case. And, if you plan to trade massages, keep your movements caressing rather than pressing. This way, you'll be able to give your partner a massage without tensing up, after you've gotten nicely relaxed from the massage you just received.

FURTHER READING

Anderson, Bob. *Stretching*. Bolinas, Ca.: Shelter Publications, 1980.

Christensen, Alice, and Rankin, David. *Easy Does It: Yoga for Older People*. Light of Yoga Society, 2134 Lee Rd., Cleveland Heights, Ohio 44118.

Furst, Jeffrey, *Over 29 Health*. Donning Publishers, 5041 Admiral Wright Rd., Virginia Beach, Va. 23462. 1979.

Kellerman, Stanley. *Your Body Speaks Its Mind*. New York: Pocket Books, 1977.

Medical Self-Care: Access to Medical Tools, a quarterly journal, P.O. Box 717, Inverness, Ca., 94937.

Mishra, R. *Fundamentals of Yoga*. New York: Lancer Books, 1959.

4.

Relaxation: The Key to Disease Resistance

WHO CAN DISPUTE THE FACT that there are mental states that lead to physical disease? Almost everyone knows people who have suffered from ulcers or heart trouble caused by too much mental and emotional pressure in their lives. These are by no means the only diseases caused by mental pressures, but they are the ones that most of us have experienced or read about.

In recent years, medical researchers have begun to employ advanced technology to explore the links between emotion and health. The study of psychosomatic medicine, of which this research is a part, is nothing new. It dates back at least as far as the fifth century to Hippocrates, who is called the father of modern medicine. Hippocrates' system of health evolved within the Greek effort to define an ideal society in which all people would find personal fulfillment and happiness. Happiness and health were synonymous, and those who were chronically unhappy invariably manifested that unhappiness with medical symptoms. Plato himself advised that one had to achieve a balance between body and mind in order to have health.

In his classic experiments on stress, Hans Selye demonstrated that emotions, such as fear and frustration, were not just ethereal experiences perceived in our brains. He showed that our experiences in life were transformed into physical changes. Some of these changes could, if prolonged, have marked effects on our overall health.*

I will never forget the first time I saw Selye's photos of glands taken from the bodies of rats placed under stress. In these photos I saw the adrenal glands of the stressed rats swollen to nearly half again their normal size, the outer membrane discolored as the result of the discharge of fatty secretion granules and stretched nearly to the bursting point, like a child's balloon. The thymus gland was a shrunken, misshapen version of its healthy counterpart. And the stomach, though not enlarged, was ulcerated and distorted.

The lymph nodes, reduced from 30 to 50 percent of their normal size, looked battered and abused, hardly capable of carrying out the complex work we depend on them to do. As useful tools, these withered little knots must have been to the doctor within what a rusty scalpel and a dull suture would be to the surgeon.

Under prolonged chronic stress, the organs that produce antibodies become shrunken, distorted, and inflamed. The production of antibodies falls dramatically, leaving the body vulnerable to infections. Temperature, moisture, and acid levels in the upper respiratory tract change, disrupting the microbial ecosystems in this area. The most prevalent infections of all—the common cold and flu and sinus infections—are likely to occur. These diseases, though usually minor, are a strain to the body, demanding work from the doctor within.

Does this mean that one scare or long period of frustration will forever cripple the immunity system? Hardly. If that were so we would all be in trouble. After periods of stress, followed by periods of relaxation, our glands regenerate themselves, just as skin regenerates itself after a cut, and antibody production returns to its normal level. However, contin-

---

* Hans Selye, *The Stress of Life,* rev. ed. (New York: McGraw-Hill, 1976).

ued stress, chronic frustration or fear, over a period of months or years, can create permanent health problems.

The Fight or Flight Syndrome

Jane Goodall, who is famous for her work with chimpanzees at the Gombe Stream Game Reserve in Tanzania, tells an interesting story of how emotions such as grief at the loss of a loved one can affect the health even of the so-called lower animals. She and her associates observed and photographed a chimpanzee named Flint after the death of his mother.

The death was a terrible shock to Flint. He had been strongly attached to his mother, who had been an important force in the chimpanzee community. He probably had a dependency on her that prevented him from easily transferring his love to another female. After her death he became withdrawn and deeply depressed. He had no appetite, and he would have little to do with other chimpanzees in the community. At last, withdrawing from all social contact, he went off alone to the last place where he had seen his mother. A short time later, Flint was found dead. An autopsy showed death had been brought on by a common virus, a virus that normally caused chimpanzees little trouble at all.* His stress and grief had reduced his resistance to disease, and so allowed the virus infection to build up into a terminal illness.

Ironically, the mechanism that causes a drop in the effectiveness of the antibody system has its roots in the ancient, inborn animal response to life-threatening situations. This is called the "fight or flight syndrome." The same mechanism that causes you to become susceptible to colds when you're under extra stress also allowed primitive man to rally his maximum physical strength when confronted by an angry tiger on a jungle trail. It is one of the paradoxes of life that this important dynamic can aid life in one situation and make it less comfortable, or even cause death, in another.

---

* Lionel Tiger, *Optimism: The Biology of Hope* (New York: Simon & Schuster, 1979).

The fight or flight syndrome works something like this: You perceive a threat and your brain automatically sends signals to two small, nondescript globs of protein attached to each of your paired kidneys. These small globs, which are actually adrenal glands, secrete hormones that your blood carries throughout your body. These hormones stimulate muscles in your arms, legs, and back, as well as your heart and lungs, enabling the muscles to act quickly and powerfully whether you decide to fight or run. One of the important things these hormones do is to cause some blood vessels to narrow and constrict blood flow while others relax and open wide. In this way the blood supply is routed for a short duration to those organs essential to immediate action, and away from those organs not essential to that action. Since the areas where antibodies are produced are not essential to running or fighting, they are temporarily robbed of nutrients, and they naturally produce fewer antibodies as a result.

The meaning of a threat is a highly individualized affair. Each one of us has a different perception of what's a threat and what isn't. Certainly, the breakup of a love affair, for example, doesn't pose the same threat to life and limb that encountering a tiger on a jungle trail might. But, for some people, the loss of love sets off events inside their bodies that cannot be distinguished from the events taking place inside the person who is facing the tiger. Similarly, it is not the work itself that causes the white-collar worker's ulcer; it is his perception of the work that counts. One person may be invigorated by the same experience, in work or play, that sends another into a wild panic.

Voodoo: The Fatality of Stress

One of the oldest and most exotic examples of the power of psychosomatic phenomena is found in the practice of voodoo. Voodoo originated in Africa as part of a religious system that focused on ancestor worship. Over the centuries, forms of voodoo have migrated to Haiti, South America, and the West Indies. Forms of it are also practiced in Australia and New Zealand.

In essence, the voodoo witch doctor casts a spell on his enemy, whereupon the enemy dies within a short period of time. In movies, Hollywood often depicts this practice as being effective regardless of the victim's walk in life. Sophisticated Westerners, raised in the cities, are shown to be just as vulnerable as the primitive tribesman who has never left the home territory of his ancestors. In real practice, this just isn't true. Voodoo spells work only on those people who strongly adhere to the total belief system in which voodoo is practiced. In other words, the spell works only if both the witch doctor and the victim are convinced it will work.

Firsthand accounts by people who have witnessed voodoo deaths describe something similar to the classic shock syndrome, familiar to every medical doctor. The victim's cheeks blanch, his eyes turn glassy and lifeless, and his facial expression becomes one either of terror or of catatonic resignation. Though the victim may make an effort to cry out, usually he can't, and the sounds choke off in his throat. He falls to the ground, his muscles twitching involuntarily. Moaning and whimpering, he covers his face with his hands and in a short while is overtaken by death.

This account provides us with some clues for a medical explanation of voodoo. The physiological mechanism goes something like this: The victim sees the witch doctor cast the spell on him, and perceives the experience as the ultimate, inescapable threat—death. Just as with the threatening perceptions that cause ulcers or stimulate hormone production, the voodoo threat is translated into physical symptoms. In voodoo, the organ affected is the heart, and this naturally has dire consequences for all other vital organs in the body.

The heart is regulated both by physical and mental impulses. An example of the *physical* impulse is when you feel your heartbeat increase during physical exercise. An example of the *mental* impulse is when you feel your heartbeat increase when you're called upon to speak before a large group of people.

The complex pumping action of the heart depends on a network of electrical impulses in various parts of the heart muscle itself. A constant rhythm of contraction and relaxation keeps blood coursing through your body to all your vital organs. As one part of the heart muscle contracts, it electrically signals another part to relax.

In a state of extreme shock, the various signals to the heart can become depressed, sending the whole blood-pumping system into a state of utter confusion. Blood pressure and blood flow drop and the entire circulatory system becomes sluggish.

Recently it has been discovered that blood clots form during extreme shock, because the flow through the blood vessels has been retarded. The clots impair or stop blood from flowing within the affected organ. When the affected organ happens to be the brain or heart, the result can be death, just as it would be with a severe heart attack or stroke.

Stress and Stomach Ulcers

Stomach ulcers offer another good example of how emotions can be converted to real physical symptoms. A stomach ulcer is created because the stomach produces too much acid (normally used to digest food), and literally causes small areas between the stomach and the upper intestine to be digested, resulting in a sore something like an abrasion or a chemical burn. Ulcers can occur elsewhere as well, but this area, the duodenum, is where stomach ulcers are most commonly found.

The overproduction of acids comes in response to certain kinds of prolonged stress. During World War II air raids in London the number of people suffering from stomach ulcers dramatically increased; the higher incidence led to our understanding the relation between stress and ulcers. In everyday life, it is the white-collar worker who most commonly suffers from an ulcer in response to a blitz of administrative demands.

There's a large nerve, called the vagus nerve, carrying signals between your stomach and your brain. When prolonged emotional pressure is experienced, whether over days or weeks or years, that pressure is translated into a signal carried by the vagus nerve to your stomach, telling your stomach to produce acids. Normally the stomach acids are produced only in the process of digesting food. In the case of the ulcer sufferer, the acids are produced not only in response to food but also in response to emotional tension. Studies have shown that even during the night, when stress would be expected to be low, and there's no food in the stomach to be digested, people with ulcers produced sixteen times more acid than people without ulcers.*

How the Mind Can Create Health

If you can accept the evidence that mental and emotional experiences can create disease, you're halfway to understanding how they can also be the source of health.

Unfortunately, having a psychosomatic illness—a disease brought on by the mind—is usually interpreted as a sign that you're weak in the head, or that your problem somehow isn't real, or even more ridiculous, that your disease is a punishment for "wrong living"! These are hardly accurate assessments of the psychosomatic (translate that as "mind-body") phenomenon. Psychosomatic diseases are, for the most part, real diseases, diseases in which actual physical events are occurring to cause discomfort, concern, and even a threat to life. Furthermore, there is abundant evidence that *most* of the diseases that plague us are either created or aggravated by mental activities. Thoughtful and forward-looking physicians are finding ways to employ this new knowledge for health.

Those physical and mental functions that make psychosomatic disease possible evolved within our bodies not to create disease but to maintain health at its optimal level. The existence of these functions is the essence of what we've called the doctor within. Creating health through them is not a matter of exerting control over them. On the contrary, it is a matter of learning to recognize when you're standing in their way, and then developing techniques to get out of their way, and to allow them to fulfill their original purpose.

---

* Arthur C. Guyton, *Textbook of Medical Physiology*, 5th ed. (Philadelphia: W. B. Saunders, 1976).

An Important Relaxation Technique

The following is an exercise that demonstrates the medical definition of relaxation and teaches you how to achieve it. By learning to consciously relax, you can restore your doctor within's capacity to guard you from infection in times of stress. The instructions are written for two participants: One person reads them while the other carries them out. If you wish to try this alone, you can do so by memorizing the instructions or by tape-recording them and playing them back.

After repeating this exercise a half-dozen times, you'll become increasingly familiar with the overall feeling of deep relaxation. Most people will then be able to induce the relaxed state simply by thinking about it, by remembering how it felt the last time they brought it on. This can be done at a desk at work, during a lunch break, or even while sitting on a bus on the way home from the office.

This exercise has several benefits in addition to those that are specifically associated with overcoming stress. It can be used to relieve everyday aches and pains in your shoulders, neck, back, and legs. In time you will see that these aches and pains are like messages being sent out by your doctor within, telling you that you need to relax. (In chapter 5, further relaxation techniques will be described as a method for overcoming chronic pain.)

INSTRUCTIONS FOR BODY RELAXATION

Lie on your back on a firm surface such as a thinly padded floor.

Let your hands rest comfortably beside you.. Your legs should be uncrossed, with heels a foot or two apart on the floor.

Your eyes should be closed.

Let your jaw go slack.

Take a deep breath. Let it out slowly.

Take a second deep breath. Let it out slowly.

Take a third deep breath. Let it out slowly.

Breathe as you normally do.

Raise your right hand, resting your elbow on the floor beside you. Make a fist. Clench it tightly. Hold it for a second or two. Let yourself concentrate on the feelings of making a fist. This is the state we call *tension*.

Relax your fist. Lower your hand gently to the floor. Imagine that arm being soft, heavy, fully released, settling comfortably against the floor. Concentrate on the feelings of your arm now. This is the state we call *relaxation*.

Repeat this with the left arm. Tense it. Note the feelings. Relax it. Note the feelings.

Tense your shoulders. Hunch them up. Hold them in the hunched position for a moment. Concentrate on these feelings of tension. Relax your shoulders. Let them be loose, sinking against the floor. Concentrate on these feelings of relaxation.

Tense your jaw muscles and simultaneously squinch up your face. Hold those positions for a moment. Note what you are feeling. These are the feelings of tension. Now relax your face and jaw muscles. Note these feelings of relaxation.

Now move down to your feet.

Tense your feet and lower legs. Hold them tense for a moment. Note the feelings. Relax them. Note the feelings of relaxation.

Tense your thigh muscles. Hold them tense for a moment. Note the feelings. Relax them. Note the feelings of relaxation.

Tense your pelvic area. Feel the muscles of your buttocks, your anus, and your genital area become tense. Hold them tense for a moment. Note the feelings of tension. Now relax the area. Note the feelings of relaxation.

Tense your stomach muscles. Hold them. Note the feelings of tension. Relax your stomach muscles. Note how they feel relaxed.

Lie flat and still for a while. Imagine your entire body sinking into the floor. Let it be heavy, soft, and, finally, fluid.

Let yourself enjoy how your body feels in this relaxed state. This is the state of full relaxation. You will feel it throughout your body, sometimes as heaviness, sometimes as tinging sensations, sometimes as feelings of warmth. These are all normal sensations of physical and mental relaxation.

When you are ready to get up, do so slowly. Let yourself be languorous and lazy for a few minutes. Then ease back into your everyday routine.

Meditation: A Release for the Healing Powers of the Doctor Within

Exhaustive research done by medical scientists has shown that during periods of deep relaxation, brain waves become slower, calmer, and more regular, allowing physiological functions to normalize. Put simply, deep relaxation allows the doctor within to work at his highest potential, free of distractions and having maximum energy. In the relaxed state, the doctor within slows heart and respiration rates, yet allows tiny blood vessels throughout your body to open, bringing an even, healthy flow of nutrients to every cell of your body. We already know that the immune system works best in the relaxed state. The healing of minor infections and the repairing of damaged tissue can also be best achieved now. Muscular, skeletal, and nerve problems—the source of many chronic pain complaints—similarly have a greater chance of mending when sufferers are relaxed.

Meditation is really nothing more than letting your mind rest while your body stays awake and alert, yet relaxed. If you have ever daydreamed—who hasn't?—or, if you have ever found your mind drifting away from your work toward a favorite recreational activity, you're already halfway to understanding what meditation is all about.

Although yogis and adherents of some of the traditional Eastern religions, such as Buddhism or Hinduism, use meditation as a way to gain spiritual understanding, we're interested here in using it to reduce the effects of stress and to enter a partnership with the doctor within.

Applications of meditation techniques run the gamut from increasing work efficiency in large corporations to aiding doctors and their patients in cancer treatment. The New York Telephone Company, in 1978, included meditation instruction as part of its regular medical program. Dr. Gilbert Callings, Jr., medical director of that company, stated that:

Results showed marked clinical improvement in reducing stress and related conditions such as irritability, depression, etc., and the most rapid improvement in these conditions came almost immediately, soon after meditation was begun.*

Learning to meditate is really very easy, but it does require some effort on the part of the beginner. The meditative state is a *normal* state of mind, one we all experience from time to time throughout our lives, whether we are aware of it or not. Why go to the bother of learning it, then? The idea is that once you can meditate at will you'll find you have gained a concrete skill or tool for comforting yourself whenever you are feeling stressed, and for cooperating with your doctor within.

The brain is accustomed to a constant flittering about of thoughts, ideas, and stimuli from the external world. In the meditative state this flittering about stops. There's an image from my past that helps me to visualize the brain's activity, and I'll pass it along to you.

When I was a boy growing up in Michigan there was an abandoned barn near my home. Most of the shingles were gone from the roof, and many boards were missing from the walls. On hot summer days it was nice to lie on the hay inside the barn and watch the endless activity of the sparrows and pigeons that lived under the eaves. When I gazed upward, I saw that the roof boards formed interstices of light and shadows against the sky. The birds flew in and out of the aging structure, weaving through the interstices, hunting insects and bits of grain, and building and repairing their nests.

When first described to me, the image of thoughts, feelings, and stimuli flittering about in the brain reminded me of the birds in the old barn. Continuing with the image, I began to perceive that the idea in meditation would be to allow thoughts, feelings, and stimuli to flitter about as they pleased, but to learn how to not follow them with the senses or be excited in any way by their movements. In other words, the idea was to realize that even though the thoughts, ideas, and stimuli continued to enter your mind, you didn't have to do anything about them. It's a bit like the first moments after en-

---

* Claire Huff, "Mantras, Meditation and Ma Bell," *San Francisco Chronicle*, September 26, 1979.

tering the barn: The birds flutter frantically, disturbed by your presence, flying from eave to eave, filling the rafters with their activity. But if you lie very still, relaxed and at ease, the activity about you slows, perhaps even ceases. Though a few random flights might occur, you would hardly be aware of them. You would notice only the clear blue sky, crosshatched by the weathered roof boards of the old barn.

It's good to remind ourselves here that meditation is not the same as daydreaming, though daydreaming is several steps in that direction. Nor is meditation a lethargic, passive state of mind. Rather, the meditative state is *focused;* while meditating, one is alert, aware, and energetic. It is interesting to note that although the meditative state is not the same as a sleep state—that is, when measured in an electroencephalogram the brain waves produced in meditation are different from those produced in sleep—people who meditate regularly report a reduction in their need for sleep.

In an electroencephalogram, the tiny electrical impulses of the brain are converted, by a machine, to lines on a piece of graph paper. A normal brain wave, one produced while you are going about your daily business, is extremely active—jagged, dense, with frequent spikes of varying heights. As you go into a meditative state, the line becomes increasingly *less* jagged, with sharp spikes being replaced by hills, valleys, and planes that are gradual and easy. A fair comparison would be something like the following:

Normal brain wave

Meditation brain wave

It is sometimes helpful to keep these graphs in mind when you are beginning to meditate and want a reference point between your normal and meditative states.

HOW TO MEDITATE

Find yourself a comfortable straight-backed chair. Sit down in it. Remove your shoes. With both your feet flat on the floor, you should feel *no* pressure on the back of your thighs where they touch the edge of the chair. If you feel pressure, put a book or two on the floor and place your feet on them, so that the weight of your legs is on the bottom of your feet rather than on the bottom of your thighs.

Loosen your belt so that you can breathe from the bottom, rather than the upper part, of your lungs. Let your hands lie in your lap, and keep your fingers, wrists, elbows, and shoulders loose and relaxed. Let your jaw drop so that your facial muscles feel loose and expressionless. Rotate your pelvis slightly forward and imagine that your spinal column, from your coccyx (tailbone) to the top of your head, is a tree growing tall and straight. You will be holding your body balanced in this position and because of that you may have to experiment with small shifts of posture before you find the position that feels right for you.

Choose a time of day and a place to meditate where you will be able to enjoy relative quiet, free of interruption, for approximately ten minutes.

First Three Days. Establish your sitting posture, as we've described above. Keep your eyes closed. Take three or four deep breaths and let your stomach expand as you do so. Let your jaw and facial muscles be relaxed. Let your shoulders, arms, and hands be relaxed.

Allowing yourself to breathe in a normal way, count your breaths. Count "one" as you breathe in. Repeat "one" as you breathe out. Count "two" as you breathe in, "two" as you breathe out, and so on.

On the first day, sit and count breaths until you reach a count of thirty-five. On the second day, increase to forty, and on the third day increase to forty-five or more if you're comfortable. An average sitting, from start to finish, will take somewhere around five minutes, though in the beginning it will probably seem much longer.

As you breathe, enjoy the subtle, sensual experience of each breath. Feel the warmth and moistness as the air moves through your air passages. Feel the slow, easy rise and fall of your chest and stomach as your lungs expand and relax.

The counting and the enjoyment of the sensations of breathing allow you to focus on the present and lead you into the meditative state. There is really nothing very mysterious about meditation; it is simply a way of focusing your attention, both mentally and physically, so that you can experience total relaxation anytime you wish.

If you are troubled by thoughts, feelings, or stimuli from the outside world, remember my image of the birds in the old barn. Imagine that your distractions are birds. Let them fly into the barn and then out of it, and remind yourself that you don't have to do anything at all about them. Remember, too, that the birds will eventually settle down or will cease to bother you.

When you've finished meditating, relax in your chair and reflect on how you feel. You may feel tingling sensations here and there, and these sensations indicate that you have learned to relax parts of your body that were previously tense. You may also notice that the world seems to have slowed down. That's because your brain waves have slowed, and as a result there are fewer signals pressing in on you, fewer things that seem to call for a response.

Surprisingly, you'll discover that you'll get more, not less, done when you start meditating regularly. With the greater focus of your attention, you waste less energy in accomplishing the things you want or need to do to make your life enjoyable and productive.

After you have finished both the meditation and your reflection, get up slowly and go about your business. As you do so, you will naturally slip into your normal daily pace. But let yourself enjoy the quieter, more relaxed, and focused meditative state from time to time throughout the day, simply by reminding yourself of how it felt while you were doing it. Just as your lips turn up in a smile when you remember something funny that happened to you in the past, so your body will relax and your mind become more focused whenever you remember how it felt the last time you meditated. The memory, of course, isn't the same as the real thing, but the more you get into the habit of regular meditation, the more the memories will provide you with numerous simulated meditations throughout the day.

Next Three Days. Start your meditation as you did for the first three days. This time, visualize a favorite subject or scene. For example, you might imagine yourself sitting quietly and peacefully at the seashore. Or you might imagine yourself on a mountain or in the desert. Or you might imagine a favorite painting or photograph that brings you feelings of inner calm.

Once you have chosen an image you like, let yourself focus on it, continuing the meditation you learned in the first three days.

At this point, you may want to extend the length of your meditation. How long you devote to it is completely up to you.

Seventh Day (and Thereafter). Start your meditation as you did for the first three days. This time imagine that you're gazing out over a distant horizon. It may be the horizon over the ocean. Or it may be a desert or forest horizon. The exact details of the image are up to you. The important part is the distant horizon.

Now imagine that your consciousness is moving slowly and gently out to the edge of the horizon. Keep your consciousness moving from your body, out to the edge of the horizon, then back to your body, over and over again, preferably following a gently flowing elliptical orbit.

Do this final meditation for ten minutes or more. Understand that the horizon, your consciousness orbiting from your body to the horizon, and even your body itself, are all being created by your mind. You are in control of everything you've imagined.

A Note on Visualization. People visualize in different ways. Some people report that they see actual pictures. Others report that they have only a vague sense of the thing taking place in their minds. Still others report an ethereal feeling that approximates what they wish to visualize. All of these forms seem to work well, so if your visualizations are less than photographic, don't be confused or frustrated. Rest assured that the kind of visualization you are having is the right one for you.

FURTHER READING

Bennett, Hal, and Samuels, Michael. *The Well Body Book*. New York: Random House, 1979.

Farquhar, John W. *The American Way of Life Need Not Be Hazardous to Your Health*. New York: Norton, 1979.

Pelletier, Kenneth R. *Mind As Healer, Mind As Slayer*. New York: Delacorte, 1977.

Rush, Anne Kent. *Getting Clear*. New York: Random House, 1973.

Selye, Hans. *The Stress of Life*. New York: McGraw-Hill, 1976.

Vickery, Donald M., and Fries, James F. *Take Care of Yourself: A Consumer's Guide to Medical Care*. Reading, Mass.: Addison-Wesley, 1976.

5.

Coping with Pain

IN RECENT YEARS, researchers have discovered that our brains produce chemicals known as *endorphins* and *enkephalins*. These chemicals, which can block pain in any part of the body, are very similar in molecular structure to such powerful opiate narcotics as heroin and morphine. Their existence was recognized in 1977, four years after scientists had discovered that specialized opiate receptor sites existed within the brain. These sites, which are located on cells, have a specific affinity for pain-relieving substances. Such drugs as morphine, heroin, Dilaudid, Talwin, Demerol, Darvon, and Percodan— all opium or opiatelike derivatives—attach themselves to opiate receptor sites to produce their effect. Because these man-made substances were readily received by sites within the body, it became clear that we each can produce our own opiatelike chemicals and that each of us is born with this ability of the brain to receive them.*

Armed with the knowledge that these substances can be created within the body, many medical researchers are now

---

* Nelson H. Hendler, and Judith A. Fenton, *Coping With Chronic Pain* (New York: Clarkson N. Potter, Inc., 1979), p. 17.

trying to discover ways of stimulating their production. Endorphins and enkephalins are seen as attractive alternatives to man-made drugs, having none of their harmful side effects. Recent tests have shown that electrical stimulation and techniques similar to acupuncture may achieve pain relief by encouraging the body to produce its own natural opiates.*

Placebos: Drugs to Stimulate Our Natural Resources

A number of experiments have demonstrated that some people produce endorphins and enkephalins when given a placebo that they're told will stop pain. Placebos, defined as "inactive substances"—in Latin, *placebo* means "I shall please"—are used routinely to test new drugs and therapies. The researcher sets up two control groups, say, Group A and Group B. Group A uses, as an example, a new caffeine and aspirin drug we will call "Painoff." Group B uses a pill that has no active ingredients whatsoever, that is, a placebo. To make certain that neither the patient nor the person administering the drugs can tell the difference between the Painoff and the placebo, both pills are made to look exactly alike. Each package of pills is given a registration number that is kept secret until the very end of the experiment. The patients receive the same instructions for the use of their pills, and such factors as patient-doctor dynamics and physical atmosphere are also the same.

When sufficient time has elapsed for the pills to have an effect, the patients are questioned about their reactions. They are not told which pills they took until the interviews have been completed. If it is discovered that there's no significant difference between Group A and Group B—that just as many patients reported benefits from the placebos as from the Painoff—it would be generally concluded that the Painoff is ineffective, or at least no more effective than the placebo. We would now suspect that these experiments provided evidence

* Ibid, p. 121.

in support of the powers of the body's own morphinelike chemicals.

In most research of this kind there is usually a significant number of patients who report dramatic benefits from the placebos. This is what's known as the "placebo effect." The patient's participation in a belief system allows the placebo to work. The patient-doctor relationship is the focus of this belief system. If the patient trusts the doctor and believes that he has the power to heal, the placebo will work better than when there is no faith in the physician. That's why a doctor's bedside manner is particularly important. A patient who feels anxious about his illness and who is suffering considerable discomfort tends to experience more relief from a placebo than one who suffers less anxiety about his illness.

Over the years, the placebo effect has been demonstrated not only in pain relievers but in everything from mild tranquilizers to the administration of antibiotics for the common cold. There are even those in the medical professions who argue that heart bypass surgery for certain angina sufferers is placebo in nature.

Shouldn't this, then, point to the work of the doctor within and teach us a deeper appreciation for the healing powers we each possess? I believe it should, and does. The placebo is a positive, health-creating influence, working within the human body to release the doctor within to do his healing work more effectively. In some respects you might look upon the placebo as a message to your doctor within to proceed with the treatment.

Pain: A Learned Response

It has long been accepted that the tolerance for pain is learned rather than inborn. Accounts by physicians working in the battlefields have reflected time and time again on how the veteran soldier is able to shut off the same degree of pain that causes inexperienced soldiers to lose consciousness. It is believed that fear of the consequences of an injury plays a role in the level of pain one experiences and that good old-fashioned stoicism can lead to shorter periods of discomfort.

But evidence suggests that the great heroes of old, who accomplished superhuman feats though painfully wounded, may not have been quite as tough as we thought they were. It is just that they had learned how to produce their own pain relievers—endorphins and enkephalins—in times of need.

Although I believe that one should be cautious about extrapolating from personal testimonies, I must say that my own experiences have supported the view of pain now being touted by medical scientists. As a child I saw my father endure constant pain from injuries he received as a soldier in World War I. He was neither a stoic nor an extraordinarily brave man. Rather, his ability to cope with pain seemed to come from a capacity to detach himself from his discomfort. It always appeared that he had a sense of humor about his pain, as if by belittling its importance he could make it go away.

The story is told in my family that my father once got into an argument with my aunt, who was a registered nurse. While she took the opposing view, my father asserted that "pain is all in your mind," and it was possible to shut it off at will. To prove his point, he had my aunt push a sterilized hatpin through the center of his hand. As the story goes, my father didn't bat an eye as the pin went through. On the contrary, he remained calm, relaxed, and even joked with others in the room as the deed was being done.

That I might have learned my father's capacity for coping with pain did not occur to me until, in my early thirties, I was injured in a motorcycle accident. I broke a number of bones, including most of the ribs in my left side, and my wrist, pelvis, and hip. All these injuries were extremely painful, as one can well imagine, but in the process I discovered that I could detach myself from pain, just as my father had done. Later, I described the experience to a friend as being something like hearing a phone ring and knowing I didn't have to answer it. The pain was definitely there. I recognized it, but I moved outside it, more like a spectator than one who was actually suffering it. Only recently have I learned to apply the same principles while in the dentist's chair, and I no longer dread my visits there.

Most large cities now have one or more pain clinics, usually sponsored by hospitals or university medical schools. The clinics work with people who suffer from chronic pain. What these clinics are proving is that people *can* be taught not simply to "tough it out" but to reduce their pain and in many cases to make it vanish altogether. In short, the doctor within is able both to administer pain relievers (endorphins and enkephalins) and reduce pain through reeducating the nervous system—with our cooperation, of course.

Some Techniques for Pain Relief

People no longer have to make a choice between enduring debilitating pain and taking drugs that often have debilitating side effects. At pain clinics, patients are taught pain relief through a number of techniques. These range from relaxation training to biofeedback training to hypnosis and even electrical nerve stimulation. As part of their program, pain clinics also offer counseling to help patients develop mental skills for dealing with the emotional difficulties that are frequently associated with pain.

Relaxation has been shown by pain clinics to be an essential means for reducing pain. Relaxing an area of your body that hurts increases blood flow to that area, bringing nutrients and pain-relieving hormones that are healing tools of the doctor within. The techniques for relaxation and meditation in chapter 4 are the basis for most of the exercises that follow.

Tension is a normal reflex that occurs whenever you injure yourself. With this tension comes a constriction of capillaries and a reduction of blood flow to the injured area. That reduced flow is important because it prevents hemorrhaging when you've cut yourself. But sometimes this mechanism doesn't stop when it should, and that prolonged tension can itself become the source of pain. Relaxation techniques then become necessary in order to signal your doctor within that it's okay to return the injured area to normal.

Some techniques, such as acupuncture and electrical nerve stimulation, are outside the scope of this book, for obvious reasons. But it is possible to describe relaxation techniques that you can do yourself without the support of pain clinics.

THE MENNINGER RX FOR HEADACHES

At the Menninger Clinic, medical researchers discovered relationships between migraine headaches and a change in the temperature of the palms. This is due to the change in the blood flow that occurs during migraine attacks.

Migraine sufferers at the Menninger Clinic were taught to go into a relaxed or meditative state and then concentrate on sensations in their hands. Electronic thermometers were taped to their palms, allowing the trainees to monitor any temperature changes they were able to create. In as few as three teaching sessions people were able to raise the temperatures in their hands several degrees. And as their palm temperatures rose, their headaches disappeared.

It is possible to learn this pain-relieving technique on your own, without an electronic apparatus to measure the temperature. First, go into a deep meditative state, using the instructions in chapter 4. Then do the following:

- Rest your hands loosely in your lap. Let your fingers be touching your palms lightly. Remember, touch lightly. Be relaxed.
- Imagine your hands are heavy, so heavy you can't lift them. Let them sink into your lap. Say to yourself, "My hands are feeling very relaxed, very, very heavy and relaxed."
- Let your neck muscles relax, too, allowing your chin to drop to your chest. Say to yourself, "My neck muscles are becoming relaxed, very loose and soft and relaxed."
- Imagine that you have two tiny hot-water bottles in your hands. Imagine that you can feel their warmth seeping into your palms. Enjoy the warmth. Feel your hands become tingly, relaxed, and warm. Imagine the heat of your palms rising two, three, four, five, even ten degrees.
- Let yourself feel and enjoy the warmth coming into your hands for several minutes. As you do this, feel your neck and shoulders relax, too.
- When you are done, return slowly to whatever it was you were doing before you started. Be at ease in your move-

ments, savoring the feelings of relaxation and warmth you experienced.

Don't be discouraged if you don't feel warmth in your palms or relief from pain the first few times you do this exercise. But keep with it. Remember that you are retraining muscles and capillaries, telling them, in essense, to give up old habits and do something that is more in tune with your doctor within.

You'll find that this headache remedy will give you relief from other discomforts as well, ranging from tooth discomfort to stiff shoulders and back pain.

ACUPRESSURE FOR HEADACHE RELIEF

Not so many years ago acupuncture was a highly charged source of controversy in the medical community. Yet now nearly every major medical facility has its resident acupuncturist, applying this ancient medical technique in a number of ways, ranging from treatment for back pain to anesthesia. We don't know exactly why acupuncture works but it is very clear that it does have some very valuable medical applications. One of the best things about it is that it has no side effects like the drugs or surgical procedures it often replaces.

Acupressure is based on the same principles as acupuncture, but since it requires no needles, you can do it yourself without the need for paraphernalia and special training. Acupressure is applied with your fingertips. You simply press on areas of your body with the padded part of your fingertips, using just the right amount of pressure to maintain a sensation that is halfway between pleasure and pain. Since you will be applying acupressure yourself in the following exercise, you can be the judge of exactly what I mean by a pressure that is halfway between pleasure and pain.

Start by sitting comfortably in a straight-backed chair. Allow yourself to be relaxed. If you wish, get into a relaxed state by following the instructions for meditation in chapter 4.

Place the padded part of your index finger in the exact center of the top of your head. Remember, apply enough pressure to get a sensation that is halfway between pleasure and pain. Now massage in slow, even circles, using only your fingertip. Make about twenty such circles, and move forward about an inch, toward your face. Again, massage in slow, even circles, using just the right amount of pressure.

Apply acupressure in the way described along every inch of the top of your head, then down your forehead to the top of your nose. When you get to your nose, use two hands. Apply pressure with your fingertips to both sides of your nose at once, applying massage in the same manner that you employed for the top of your head. Work down along your face, around your mouth to the bottom of your jaw.

Finish up by applying the same acupressure technique to your temples, being especially careful here to apply just the right amount of pressure.

When done, let your hands lie relaxed in your lap. Let your head and face tingle for a few moments—they will if you've applied the fingertip acupressure in the way I've described—and let yourself be aware of and enjoy these sensations.

This treatment is especially helpful for headache and facial pain associated with colds and sinus infections. But it can be equally effective for most tension headaches.

The same techniques used here can be applied to other kinds of pain that might occur anywhere in your body. The book on acupressure noted at the end of this chapter will show you how to use acupressure for specific problems.

A RECORDED MESSAGE FOR DEEP MUSCLE RELAXATION

To further experience your potential for learning to be free of pain, try this exercise. Read the following sentences into a tape recorder. Read in a slow, metered, soothing voice. Then relax yourself or meditate. Once in your relaxed state, play back your tape and follow the instructions you've given yourself.

1. You are feeling relaxed and comfortable, very still in your mind. You feel comfortable and open.

2. Without moving other areas of your body, clench your fist. Make your fist as hard as you can. Hold it in a hard fist for fifteen or twenty seconds.

3. Suddenly release your fist. Open your hand and let it lie loose and limp in your lap.

4. Focus your attention on your hand and arm. What sensations do you feel? Explore these sensations. Feel them. Experience them.

5. Make a hard fist again. What sensation do you feel now? Explore these sensations. These are the sensations of tension.

6. Suddenly relax your wrist. Explore the feelings in your hand and arm. These are the feelings of relaxation.

7. Clamp your jaw muscles tightly, as though gritting your teeth against pain. Hold your jaw tight for ten seconds. This is tension. Release your jaw. Let your mouth hang open. These are the sensations of relaxation.

8. Hunch up your shoulders as you would to ward off the cold. Hold them tight for a few seconds. Explore the sensations of tension you now feel. Suddenly drop your shoulders. Let them be loose. Explore these sensations of relaxation.

9. Exhale. Empty your lungs. Now tighten the muscles of your stomach. As you do this, other muscles of your torso will tighten. Explore these sensations of tension. Let your muscles relax. Let your lungs fill slowly, as though you were filling a bottle of water at a spring. Breathe slowly and easily. Explore the sensations of your relaxed torso.

10. Clamp your knees together. Release them. Clamp them together again and hold them for ten or fifteen seconds. Explore these sensations of tension. Suddenly relax your knees. Explore these sensations of relaxation.

11. Curl up your toes. Hold them tightly curled. Explore these feelings of tension in your feet and calves. Release your toes. Explore these feelings of having your feet completely relaxed.

12. Quickly do the following. Tense and release your fists. Tense and release your jaw. Tense and release your shoulders. Exhale. Tense and release your stomach. Inhale slowly. Clamp your knees together. Release them. Curl your toes. Release them.

13. Sit for ten or fifteen seconds and explore the sensations of being relaxed all over.

14. If you feel tension in an area of your body, tense the muscles of that area. Relax them. Tense and relax them several times until the area feels loose and open.

This exercise teaches you, on a subliminal, or kinesthetic level, how it feels to relax your muscles deeply, and how it feels to make them tense. The knowledge, recorded in your body, allows you to tell any area you wish to relax. Each time you repeat this exercise, the kinesthetic knowledge goes deeper and deeper, and you gain strength in your ability to open your body to the healing tools of your doctor within.

ZEN PAIN RELIEF

With any tool, it's a good idea to learn how to operate it smoothly before you need to use it. This certainly holds true for techniques for relieving pain. The following tool is presented in steps—beginning, intermediate, and advanced— so that you can master it and have it on hand.

The beginning step, which is focused on a ringing telephone, may seem unrelated to pain. But consider this: The senses with which you hear the ringing phone, as well as your associations with who may be trying to reach you, all take place inside you. In the final analysis, there are strong parallels between the ringing phone and pain. If this isn't comprehensible to you right away, be assured that it will be by the time you've mastered all three steps of this exercise.

You may be interested in knowing the sources of these exercises. The intermediate and advanced steps—those that deal with itching and pain—are techniques that will be familiar to most students of Zen Buddhism. The young monk is required to sit for long periods of time, sometimes for hours each day, as he learns the rigors of meditation. The usual aches, pains, and itches to which we normally respond must be ignored. A swat on the head by the Zen Master is the monk's reward for wiggling when he should be meditating. Thus, young monks are taught the techniques I describe here, in order that their discipline will not be interrupted by the mundane signals of the flesh. Similar techniques are being applied at pain clinics.

The beginning step, the ringing telephone, is, as far as I know, my own invention.

Beginning. The next time your telephone rings, don't answer it. Probably your mind will become active as the ringing continues. You may be curious about who's calling you. You may find yourself wondering if you are needed by someone in trouble. You may wonder if you're passing up a golden opportunity. Or you may feel sociable and start imagining how nice it would be to have someone to talk to. To answer a ringing phone is a powerful temptation. Still, let it ring. Concentrate on the sound of the bell, and the quality of the ringing. Allow your curiosity about who might be on the other end to fade away as you explore the qualities of the *sound* of the ringing phone.

Intermediate. The next time you get that aggravating back itch that you can't quite reach, take advantage of the opportunity to practice this technique: Let yourself feel the itch. Say to yourself, "Itching. Itching. Itching." Examine the quality of the itch. Really let yourself get into it, just as though you were listening to a fine bell being rung in a church steeple. Let yourself admire its clarity and persistence, but do nothing else about it. After a few moments, imagine that your doctor within is assuming responsibility for the itching signal. Tell yourself that he is taking care of the matter and that you no longer have to do anything about it.

Advanced. Most of us suffer minor injuries from time to time, such as hitting our thumb with a hammer or catching a finger in the door, or stubbing a toe on the nightstand. Next time any of these happens to you, practice the same principles you learned in mastering the itch or letting the phone ring. Sit down, relax as much as you can, and say, "Pain. Pain. Pain." to yourself, over and over again. Examine the qualities of the pain signal until you decide to turn the matter over to your doctor within.

If a cut or a broken bone is involved, first do whatever you can do at that moment to take action to aid the healing. This can mean anything from putting on a Band-Aid to getting someone to drive you to the doctor. At the point when you feel confident that you have done everything that needs to be done, turn your attention to mastering the pain, just as you have learned to do above. Be confident in your ability to develop this tool. It works.

NAME THAT PAIN

Perhaps after doing the foregoing exercises you've found yourself turning more attention to the specific area of your body where you frequently feel pain. Your reflex may be to pay much attention to the pain at the same time that you're making an effort to somehow escape from it. A part of you really wants to deny its existence.

According to many authorities on pain, this effort to deny its existence becomes, in effect, a source of anxiety, and increases tension and pain. There has been a good deal of success in reducing pain by zeroing in on this very mechanism in our lives.

Many pain clinics ask people to focus right in on their pain. They instruct pain sufferers to scrutinize the qualities of their pain with the same critical eye with which they would scrutinize a character in a novel, movie, or theater production. They are asked to begin this critical examination by assigning words to their pain. Here is a partial list of sample descriptive words: dull, aching, tender, splitting, throbbing, stabbing, grueling, cruel, crushing, flashing, prickling, sharp, gnawing, searing, fearsome, blinding, pressing, gripping, tugging, demanding. Although this list is not comprehensive, it should give you a place to start. What happens is that as you explore and then name your pain, you begin to demystify it. As this happens, anxiety about it is reduced, and at least that level of the pain experience is diminished.

Naming the qualities of one's pain brings that pain into the realm of the manageable. Our minds, after all, have a way of creating a distance between ourselves and our fears as soon as we assign names to those fears. The same mechanism can work with chronic pain.

BIOFEEDBACK TRAINING

If the present level of research in biofeedback training continues, this form of therapy will one day replace hundreds of pharmaceuticals and surgical procedures. What exactly is biofeedback training? *Biofeedback* simply means the signals that make you become consciously aware of a physiological change in your body. When you feel tension in your hand and forearm while making a fist, that's biofeedback. On a more complex level, a biofeedback therapist might fasten a temperature sensor to the palm of your hand and hook it up to a machine that would show you, with a light or a sound, whenever the temperature in your hand goes up or down.

The purpose of biofeedback training is to teach people to voluntarily control bodily functions that were previously thought to be involuntary. It has been found that many diseases are caused by small errors in our daily functions, such as too much stomach acidity, or tension in a muscle or a group of muscles that should be relaxed. Usually these errors are learned at an early age. Most people who complain of chronic headaches, for example, have unconsciously learned to tense muscle tissue in their necks and shoulders in response to stressful experiences, a response that might be compared to the reflex of *ducking* when someone takes a swipe at you.

Because they've learned this so early in life, these reflexes become automatic and seem natural or normal to them by the time they reach adulthood. When asked if they feel any tension in their neck and shoulders, many headache sufferers answer no. The tense state has become so much a part of their lives that they're not conscious of what they do to produce it. But when electronic instruments are applied to measure muscular tension, these people can see that they are indeed tensing up. Using the same machine as a monitor, they are shown how to relax these muscles and bring permanent freedom from chronic headaches.

Muscle tension is only one of several functions we can monitor with modern biofeedback instruments. We can also measure respiration and heart rates, the acid levels of any organ in the body, and nerve impulses carrying messages to and from the brain to any specific area of the body.

One of the first questions people ask about biofeedback training is whether or not such controls over our bodily functions are dangerous. Extensive research has been done on this question. Because of the techniques involved, harming yourself through biofeedback training is virtually impossible. The training is based on relaxing rather than exerting control over physiological functions. In effect, you let go of controlling factors that have caused disease and allow your doctor within to restore those functions to a healthy level.

A typical biofeedback training session might go something like this: Half a dozen people sit at small tables in an ordinary classroom. On the table in front of each person is an instrument that looks like a transistor radio. The class is instructed to tape two simple heat sensors to the palms of their hands.

The teacher now reads instructions for the students to go into a deeply relaxed, meditative state. Once relaxed, the students are asked to imagine the temperature of their palms going up. They are asked nothing more: just relax and imagine the temperature of your palms rising.

After a few moments, first one and then another of the instruments on the students' desks give off gentle humming sounds, which signal that the students have succeeded in raising the temperature of their palms.

The students are told to make a note of how they feel when the signal is heard. They are told that after several sessions they'll be able to accomplish the same thing without the aid of their electronic instruments, by learning to reproduce the experience of raising their palm temperatures.

Palm temperature is affected by relaxing neck and shoulder muscles. As one relaxes these muscles, blood flow to the palms as well as to the head returns to a normal level. By concentrating on their palms, people automatically release the muscles in their shoulders and neck, bringing about the relief they seek.

In addition to overcoming chronic pain, biofeedback techniques have proved valuable in teaching people how to regain motor control after stroke, and how to regain muscular control with many forms of paralysis and spasticity after damage to the nervous system through disease or injury. Facial tics and the loss of control over facial muscles following the severance of a nerve have also been successfully treated with biofeedback training.

Promising treatment techniques with biofeedback are beginning to be developed for a wide range of medical problems—angina, Raynaud's disease (a disease affecting blood flow in the hands and feet), bronchial asthma, insomnia, eczema, neurodermatitis, palsy, hyperactivity in children, and even glaucoma. There are some interesting experiments that have demonstrated as well that birth control may one day be learned through biofeedback. To accomplish this, men learn to raise the temperature of their scrotum, which reduces their levels of sperm production for a short period of time. Similarly, women are able to voluntarily change the acid levels of their vaginas, making fertilization impossible.

Probably the most important message biofeedback training has for all of us is that medical researchers are beginning to develop effective techniques for treating our illnesses without the need for radical invasive surgery or drugs that in themselves have posed threats to health. Here is one area of medicine in which the powers to heal are being returned to the doctor within, whose wisdom and power to heal is vastly broader than our best-trained medical teams.

Resources for More Pain Relief

The following are professional societies that can help you either find more literature about freeing yourself from pain or can direct you to nearby clinics where you can get direct help.

Arthritis Foundation
3400 Peachtree St., NE
Atlanta, GA 30326

Biofeedback Society of America
University of Colorado Medical Center
Denver, CO 80260

American Association for the Study of Headache
5252 N. Western Ave.
Chicago, IL 60625

National Migraine Foundation
2422 W. Foster Ave.
Chicago, IL 60626

International Association for the Study of Pain
Dept. of Anesthesiology
University of Washington
Seattle, WA 98195

American Association for the Advancement of Tension
Control
P.O. Box 8005
Louisville, KY 40208

FURTHER READING

Chan, Pedro. *Finger Acupressure.* New York: Ballantine Books, 1976.

Feuerstein, Michael, and Skjei, Eric. *Mastering Pain.* New York: Bantam Books, 1979.

Fryling, Vera, and Halpern, Steven. *Autogenic Training.* (Recorded cassette tape of instructions.) Autogenics, 2510 Webster St., Berkeley, Ca. 94205.

Hendler, Nelson H., and Fenton, Judith A. *Coping with Chronic Pain.* New York: Clarkson N. Potter, 1979.

Shealy, C. Norman. *Ninety Days to Self-Health.* New York: Dial, 1977.

6.

The Healing Powers of Sleep and Dreams

EACH YEAR RESEARCHERS DISCOVER more about sleep. Most of the research comes down to this: Sleep puts the body and mind on a holding pattern, allowing the doctor within to catch up with the work that has accumulated during our waking hours. As we sleep the doctor within hangs out his shingle and gets down to work.

When we are deprived of sleep for long periods, even the smallest routine tasks begin to seem like high-stress confrontations. We get jumpy, irritable, and short of temper. Our appetite may diminish altogether or be expressed in strange food cravings at strange times. We find ourselves mentally distracted, making mistakes, and unable to concentrate. Deprived of sleep for long enough, we begin to hallucinate, imagining people and objects that aren't really there, just as though we were dreaming while awake. Our mental and emotional lives suffer, and our bodies suffer as a result.

Most people look upon sleep as a totally passive state, a period during which nothing much is happening. It may be that we stop interacting with the external world during this time, but events continue to take place inside us that are no less important than those that take place in the external world.

During sleep the pituitary gland releases growth hormones. These hormones are associated with a deep sleep state in which the brain waves become very slow and relaxed. In children the hormones are important because they stimulate bone growth. In adults, though less important, these hormones play an essential role in the renewal processes in bones and in the production of blood cells within the bones.

Adrenal hormones (a group known as hydroxycorticosteroids) are also secreted in the deepest stages of sleep. These hormones are important in the digestion of proteins and fats and in the production of glucose in the blood, which supplies the cells with their energy. Without these hormones you would be unable to resist physical or mental stress, and even minor infections could become fatal. Experiments have shown that we have the highest levels of these hormones in our bloodstream in the first few hours after waking, and the lowest just before retiring at night.

Scientists don't yet understand all the healing properties of sleep but there is no doubt that the doctor within makes good use of this time. One hint we have is that during sleep the production of new cells in the mucosal tissue of our mouths, to replace cells damaged by trauma, infection, and age, goes on at a much more rapid rate than in our waking hours. It is very possible that researchers in the future will be able to demonstrate that similar increased healing rates occur elsewhere in the human body as we sleep.

One physiologist* describes sleep as a "rezeroing" of the body and mind—using the analogy of the computer which after prolonged use must be shut down and rezeroed in order to renew its baseline of operations. The basis for this theory is that as we sleep our arterial blood pressure drops, our pulse rate decreases, skin vessels dilate, and muscles throughout our bodies become completely relaxed. Our overall metabolic rate goes down 10 to 20 percent. Similarly, activity within our nervous system slows, as illustrated in the electroencephalo-

---

* Arthur C. Guyton, *Textbook of Medical Physiology*, 5th ed. (Philadelphia: W. B. Saunders, 1976).

graph samples on the next page. Although brain activity continues in the deep sleep state, it is considerably diminished, as a comparison of the two graphs quickly demonstrates.

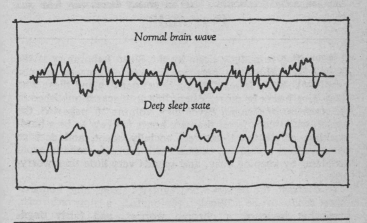

Normal brain wave

Deep sleep state

How the Rhythms of Sleep Affect Your Mood

There is a sleep pattern that all of us who are in good health follow. We go from light sleep to deep sleep and back again to light sleep in approximately ninety-minute cycles. During parts of each cycle we go into a state of consciousness that researchers call REM, or Rapid Eye Movement, sleep. REM is the period during which we dream.

If you are deprived of the REM periods of sleep, you soon become moody and anxious, and you find it difficult to concentrate. Muscular coordination goes awry and cardiovascular rhythms are disrupted. In experiments in which animals were deprived of REM sleep, they eventually became mentally deranged, returning to normal only after they were able to catch up on their lost sleep. The sleep induced by sleeping pills is not desirable for this reason. In addition to the fact that they are frequently addictive and become ineffective after a few weeks of use, sleeping pills rob the sleeper of REM sleep.

How Your Sleep Habits May Reflect Your Personality

According to a study done by the Sleep Laboratory at the Boston State Hospital, there are marked differences between people who sleep fewer than six hours per day and those who sleep nine hours or more. According to a report published in the *Archives of General Psychiatry*, volume 26, page 463, the person who sleeps fewer than six hours is likely to be a hard-working, efficient, self-assured, socially adept, and decisive person. He is ambitious, content with himself, tends to avoid problems by keeping busy, and spends very little time worrying.

In contrast, the person who regularly sleeps nine hours or more tends to be critical, opinionated, a nonconformist, somewhat insecure, a chronic worrier, and fairly unaggressive. He may be overtly anxious, and somewhat inhibited sexually.

How Your Work Efficiency Is Affected by Sleep

According to surveys, about half the American population over fifteen years of age complains of suffering from some form of sleeplessness at least once in their lives. About 15 percent of our nation's population complains of having chronic sleep problems, and about 33 percent say they have recurrent experiences with insomnia. Here are some interesting facts about insomnia:

- Insomniacs take longer to fall asleep than people with more normal sleep patterns.
- After finally getting to sleep, insomniacs awaken during the

night about the same number of times as normal sleepers, but while the normal sleeper later has no recollection of awakening, the insomniac remembers every moment awake.

- Insomniacs dream more than normal sleepers.
- Insomniacs tend to obtain less deep sleep (known as "stage IV" sleep) than normal sleepers.

And how is your efficiency affected by the loss of sleep? Here are some more facts:

- After 36 hours of continuous work with no sleep, efficiency declines by 15 percent.
- After 44 hours of continuous work with no sleep, efficiency declines by 20 percent.
- After 48 hours of continuous work with no sleep, efficiency declines by 35 percent.
- After 36 hours of continuous work with no sleep, there is a 58 percent recovery of efficiency after only 2 hours of sleep.
- After 36 hours of continuous work with no sleep, there is a 73 percent recovery of efficiency after 4 hours of sleep.
- After 36 hours of continuous work with no sleep, there is a full recovery of work efficiency after 12 hours of sleep.

Improving Your Sleep

Sometimes people overlook the obvious when it comes to solving sleep problems. For example, make certain that your mattress is comfortable, and that the room in which you sleep is at a comfortable temperature. If sex relaxes you, keep that in mind as a natural sleep inducer. However, people who feel active and energetic after sex should seek other relaxants to coax them to sleep.

People's sleep needs are as individual as their appetites and consciences. If you're troubled because you can't seem to get more than six hours of sleep at night, ask yourself if you really need any more than that. The main issue here is, how do you feel in the morning? Do you feel rested and ready to start the day even though you've slept only six hours? If so, you're getting the right amount of sleep for you. If, however, you awaken feeling tired and without energy, consider the suggestions below.

SLEEP REMEDIES

Cut out all caffeine: *Coffee, black tea, cola drinks, chocolate, many cold pills, and many headache remedies contain this drug. Some people will argue that these things never bothered them before, so why should they bother them now? Recent research reveals that the older we get the less tolerance we have for caffeine, and the more powerfully it acts upon our system.*

Avoid recreational drugs: *Alcohol and marijuana can inhibit REM sleep or cause you to awaken early.*

Drink warm milk before retiring: *The effective ingredient of this folk remedy has recently been found to contain L-triptophan, a substance naturally produced by our bodies that induces drowsiness. Meat and green vegetables also contain this substance in significant amounts.*

Drink camomile tea before retiring: *This tea has long been recognized for its soothing effect, even though no research has been done to reveal its active ingredient. Available at health food stores and some supermarkets.*

Meditation: *Use the instructions contained in chapter 4. Meditation empties your mind and relaxes your muscles, and these are the first steps toward sleep.*

Light exercise: *If you are not getting aerobic exercise on a regular basis, try walking for a mile or so before retiring at night. Your muscles will relax and you'll lie down with a feeling of well-being that will carry you toward sleep.*

Psychotherapy: *Many people find that night after night they lie awake trying to solve problems they're having with other people in their lives. Working with a good psychotherapist provides them with tools for solving these problems instead of letting them cause insomnia.*

The Function of Dreaming

Dreams are a normal part of sleep, and although we rarely remember them upon waking, research shows that they are universally experienced. Everyone dreams and everyone reaps the benefits of this mental activity. Like sleep, dreams affect our physical health through our minds.

In the early 1900s the psychologist C. G. Jung urged people to look past the two popular views that then prevailed—that dreams were the work of Satan or that they were the result of indigestion. Jung believed that dreams were created from the material we store in our minds and were an important health factor in our lives. According to Jung, dreams reflect the *unconscious* mind, wherein everyday experiences and wishes, dating back perhaps as far as our life in the womb, are stored in a sort of poetic form in our minds. With a language rich in imagery and symbolism, it is as if their maker—the doctor within?—has deliberately compressed them into well-hewn artifacts. Jung said: "The unconscious is not a demonic monster but a thing of nature that is perfectly neutral as far as moral sense, aesthetic taste and intellectual judgment go."*

Working with his own dreams and the dreams of his patients and fellow doctors, Jung discovered that two essential human needs were fulfilled through the poetry of the unconscious: The first was that dreams provided a way to store the experiences the dreamer collected throughout his life; the second was that dreams provided the dreamer with a way to compensate for things that he couldn't do or had more sense than to do in real life. In their compensatory form, dreams could run the gamut from the adolescent's dream of sexual fulfillment to the adult's dream of domination over a tyrannical authority figure.

The compensatory needs of the human animal are acted out in many ways other than dreams, of course. For example,

---

* C. G. Jung, "Dream-Analysis in Its Practical Application," from *The Basic Writings of C. G. Jung* (New York: Modern Library, 1959).

we read books, or go to movies where we become immersed in high adventure and intrigue. We momentarily identify with heroes and heroines who are doing dangerous or violent things, and we enjoy these bizarre exaggerations of real life not because we're violent and bloodthirsty ourselves but, on the contrary, because we aren't. What, then, is the wellspring that causes us to develop this taste for exciting events unlike those that occur in our daily lives?

Civilized living requires constant compromises and reasonable negotiations that leave ragged edges of frustration even when we feel that our decisions to compromise or negotiate have been justified and fair. Our capacity for dreaming provides us with a theater for acting out feelings that if acted out in real life could prove dangerous, unfair to our loved ones, or just plain embarrassing. As a tool for the doctor within, dreams provide a safety valve for blowing off psychological steam.

C. G. Jung believed that dreams were important to health, that the ability to dream was one of the body's ways of maintaining balance and harmony between all its various parts. In speaking of our mental and emotional life he hypothesized that the unconscious mind, and dream, constituted:

> . . . a self-regulating system that maintains itself in equilibrium as the body does. Every process that goes too far immediately and inevitably calls forth a compensatory activity. Without such adjustments a normal metabolism would not exist, nor would the normal psyche.*

KEEPING A DREAM DIARY

Since dreams are the tools of the doctor within, it is important to remember, record, and interpret them. Whatever insights dreams may give you into yourself, they are a normal function of the self-healing systems that were built into your body at birth. A dream diary can help.

Get yourself a small notebook, such as a steno pad, and keep it beside your bed at night. When you awaken each morning spend a few minutes before arising to make notes

---

* Ibid.

about your dreams. If you can't remember any dreams, make an entry saying so. If you can remember only a fragment of a dream, write that down. The important thing is to make a habit of writing something in your dream diary each time you awaken. You'll be surprised how, by establishing this habit in your life, you automatically begin to recall your dreams in detail.

As you record your dreams, resist the temptation to censor or interpret them. Record them with the objectivity with which you snap a photograph. Remember what Jung said about dreams being neutral, and allow that insight to guide you. Don't be dismayed if your dreams express things which in real life you would never, for a moment, seriously entertain. Thinking or imagining a thing in no way implies you will one day do it. Stop to consider this—that if dreaming did work that way, every driveway would have a Porsche, Rolls-Royce, Mercedes Benz, or similar car parked in it.

Most psychologists agree that dreams, like poetry, are constructed with a highly personalized language, imagery, and symbolism. A few dream symbols—very few!—do seem to be universal *most* of the time, but a too liberal interpretation is seldom helpful.

How does one make any useful sense of dreams? Look for situations and themes that repeat themselves. For example, let's say that after several weeks of recording your dreams you notice that you dream about conflicts with people who consistently make you feel helpless. Ask yourself if this experience correlates with anything in your real life: a bossy parent, a pushy employer, a domineering mate, or even a spoiled son or daughter. You'll usually discover parallels between your real life and your dream life. Recognize that dreams are a means of searching for better methods of handling difficult situations in your life. Let this knowledge direct your path toward books, friends, professional counselors, or classes through which you can learn more effective skills for handling the specific kinds of conflicts your dreams define.

The dream diary, like a mirror, will reflect an image of who you are. Becoming familiar with your inner life as reflected in your dreams, need require very little more "reasonable" effort on your part than looking at yourself in the mirror each morning. Many kinds of important self-knowledge can be gained only by observing without judging ourselves.

FURTHER READING

Horney, Karen. *Our Inner Conflicts.* New York: Norton, 1966.

Luce, Gay Gaer. "Current Research on Sleep and Dreams." U.S. Department of Health, Education and Welfare, National Institute of Mental Health, Public Health Service Publication 1389 (1965).

McLeester, Dick. *Welcome to the Magic Theatre: A Handbook for Exploring Dreams.* Food for Thought Publications, Box 331, Amherst, Mass., 01002.

Thoresen, Carl E., and Coates, Thomas J. *How to Sleep Better: A Drug-Free Program for Overcoming Insomnia.* Englewood Cliffs, N.J.: Prentice-Hall, 1977.

Walker, C. Eugene. *Learn To Relax: 13 Ways to Reduce Tension.* Englewood Cliffs, N.J.: Prentice-Hall, 1975.

7.

Physical Conditioning for the Well Body

THERE IS A GROWING BELIEF in the medical community that the human body is simply not suited to the sedentary life-style of the twentieth century. The differences in attitude, body chemistry, immune system responses, bone and muscle consistency, and in the cardiovascular systems, between the person who gets exercise and the person who doesn't is vast. A person in good physical condition not only seems to have greater resistance to disease but he also seems to recover more rapidly from disease and injury than those who are sedentary.

In the not so distant past the accepted course of treatment for a patient who had suffered a heart attack was inactivity and bedrest. Usually, the heart attack victim sat around the house, depressed, anxious, and filled with feelings of uselessness. Between stress and inactivity, he was lucky to survive the next five years.

Now the picture is changing. In many cases, heart attack victims are put on an exercise program within a matter of days after their attack. Of course, this is not done without caution. The patient may undergo many tests, including a stress test in which his heart capacities are monitored as he works out on a treadmill. After the limits are established, an exercise program is designed for the patient. Once he begins the program, his progress is monitored by frequent checkups.

People in good physical condition have a larger capacity for stress of all kinds—physical, emotional, and intellectual. It is believed that this is related to the increase in nutrients that each cell (brain and body alike) is able to assimilate. It is also related to certain hormonal events that occur in your body when you exercise.

During exercise, the adrenal hormones become particularly active. At least one of these hormones, *norepinephrine*, has profound effects on the emotions. Research shows that this hormone—which is secreted when the body is pressed into action—acts as a mood elevator, more powerful than any of the drugs that chemists have created for that same purpose. Anyone who is jogging regularly will have experienced "runner's high," a sense of well-being and mild euphoria triggered by the body's sending shots of this hormone into the bloodstream.

At Purdue University, Dr. A. H. Ismail tested the chemical changes in the bodies of a group of middle-aged college professors before and after a five-month jogging program. He found that even moderate running changed glucose and testosterone levels. He also found a marked reduction in the bloodstreams of substances called *catecholamines*, which are known to be associated with states of aggression, anxiety, and depression. The researcher stated that after only ten weeks, his subjects began to undergo subtle but definite personality changes: "They became more open and extroverted. And their whole demeanor seemed more stable and self-confident."*

That physical exercise strengthens your antibody system should seem obvious when you stop to consider that the production of antibodies and the delivery of those antibodies to the sites of infection are largely accomplished through the blood. Consider, further, that blood flow is vastly increased by a regular exercise program. People literally grow more

---

* Valerie Andrews, *The Psychic Power of Running* (New York: Ballantine Books, 1979).

blood vessels when they exercise regularly, guaranteeing an increased blood supply—with its antibodies—to all areas of their bodies.

Regular exercise causes your body to secret large quantities of the hormone norepinephrine. This hormone helps your antibody system indirectly by releasing certain white blood cells that ordinarily cling to the walls of blood vessels. The hormone causes them to become very active and to circulate freely, reducing infection in their wake.

At the same time that norepinephrine is being released, its companion hormone, *epinephrine*, flows through your body. This hormone increases your metabolic rates as much as 100 percent. Heart rate and blood flow, carrying white blood cells and antibodies, become vastly more effective.

Physical exercise requires heavy breathing, and with this comes a stimulation of the mucosal blanket that coats and protects your respiratory tract. Antibodies are present in this blanket and become increasingly effective as it becomes more moist and active with exercise.

Finally, exercise allows your body to relax in ways that might otherwise be impossible. Hormones released during exercise continue to have an effect for a number of hours. These hormones, plus substances produced in your muscle tissue while exercising, induce a sense of well-being and relaxation, a physiological state that is not unlike the meditative state we described in chapter 4. As you'll recall, this meditative state is both mental and physical, increasing blood flow to all areas of the body associated with the production of antibodies.

Exercise as a Cure for Cancer

In establishing the relationships between stress and disease, Dr. Hans Selye postulated that exercise may actually help the body cure cancer by providing a way to release tension. Because stress reduces antibody activity, the speculation that exercise might increase it through reducing stress would seem reasonable. It has also been speculated by medical scientists that stress makes the body more susceptible to cancer, so exercise can in fact be seen as preventive medicine to protect you from ever getting the disease.

Dr. O. Carl Simonton, director of the Simonton Center for Cancer Counseling and Research in Forth Worth, Texas, has also done research on exercise and tumor reduction. Although it is too early to draw any conclusions, some of the stories of his successes are promising. He tells of one patient who completed the Honolulu Marathon run even though he was being treated for lung cancer. After the race the runner felt healthy, happy, and full of energy, looking forward to a full future. Although nothing is proved by such physical feats, Simonton has been able to establish that exercise programs help cancer patients develop new trust in their bodies and develop a greater sense of hope and self-esteem.

In addition to their physical training, patients at Simonton learn to meditate and visualize cancer cells as weak, second-rate invaders of a strong body. They receive instruction in specific areas of stress reduction, and in resolving long-standing emotional conflicts in their lives.

In his research Dr. Simonton has demonstrated that rates of recovery from cancers previously diagnosed as terminal are highest among those patients who have good feelings about their bodies. In marked contrast, the patients with lowest rates of recovery are those who feel overwhelmed by their disease and think of their bodies as "the enemy."

The record at the Simonton clinic, based on 159 patients with what had been diagnosed as incurable cancer (usual life expectancy about twelve months), showed that 40 percent were living active lives two years later. Seven out of ten of those either had complete cures or their tumors were regressing. Overall, the Simonton clinic's combined treatment techniques result in cure rates nearly twice as good as traditional medical treatment such as surgery, chemotherapy, and cobalt, alone.

Regular Physical Exercise: Working Miracles in the Cardiovascular System

Probably the most dramatic changes from regular physical exercise occur in the cardiovascular system. According to Kenneth H. Cooper, the aerobics expert, an average man with good physical conditioning will carry as much as a quart more blood than the same size man who is not well conditioned.

When you stop to consider that the heart is a muscle, one that requires blood flow in the same way as the arms and legs, the prescription for exercise seems logical. Leg and arm muscles increase in strength with use, decrease with nonuse. Exercise increases blood flow, makes arteries more flexible and strong, and even encourages the growth of new blood vessels.

The larger blood supply and growth in the arterial system provide an increased blood flow to every cell in the body. Also, the increase in the strength and capacity of the cardiovascular system means that more oxygen is being supplied to all cells, for the simple reason that an increase in red blood cell circulation provides an increase in oxygen uptake.

At the Cardiac Rehabilitation Unit at Los Amigos Hospital in Downey, California, doctors have been working with heart attack victims for several years. Most of the participants in the program have recovered from their heart attacks, and have gone on to enjoy a higher level of health than they had before the attack. Runners who started exercising in order to get well again have developed into real athletes, though they had never been particularly athletic before. Many patients have taken up bicycle riding—an activity that is particularly encouraged—and are riding in "centuries"—organized rides of 100 miles in a day. Stories of heart attack victims becoming marathon runners or even "triple century" (300 miles in a day) bike riders are not at all unusual.

The literature of the medical establishment is often very cautious in stating trends in new treatments, but careful readings will reveal what those trends might be. In the recent edition of *The Merck Manual** (ordinarily a conservative reference for doctors), the authors state that after a satisfactory six-week recovery period following a heart attack, most patients are able to return to their full range of normal activity and "some established more regular exercise programs than prior [to their attacks]."

Most doctors recommend that if you're over forty and have not been exercising regularly but are in good health, you should work with your physician to tailor an exercise program for you. The cardiovascular system builds up quickly—within two or three months in most cases—but because of our sedentary life-styles we may have abused our bodies enough to require some gentle coaxing at first. In large cities there are usually cardiologists who offer complete testing and guidance for people who wish medical consultation in starting their exercise programs. In many cities there are also complete cardiovascular programs sponsored by such groups as the YMCA, which help a wide range of people with special problems, guiding even those who have suffered heart attacks into regular, vigorous physical exercise. It should be recognized that there really are no age limits for this. More and more people in their sixties, seventies, and even eighties are beginning to exercise regularly.

A TEST FOR PHYSICAL CONDITIONING

Here is an easy test you can give yourself before you begin a regular exercise program.

Preparation. Sit quietly for five minutes or more. Then take your pulse, by counting pulse beats at your wrist, or by counting them at the carotid artery. See illustration opposite.

Count your heartbeats for a full sixty seconds. Sixty beats, or fewer, per minute is very good. That means you're in good condition. Eighty beats or more per minute means you aren't in such good shape, and you could benefit greatly from a reg-

---

* *The Merck Manual of Diagnosis and Therapy,* 13th ed. (Rahway, N.J.: Merck & Co., Inc., 1977).

ular exercise program. Seventy to seventy-five beats is about average.

CHOOSING THE RIGHT EXERCISE PROGRAM

For the kinds of benefits we're discussing here, regular, evenly paced exercise is better than exercise that stops and starts. For example, twenty minutes of straight, even jogging without stops provides you with more aerobic benefit than

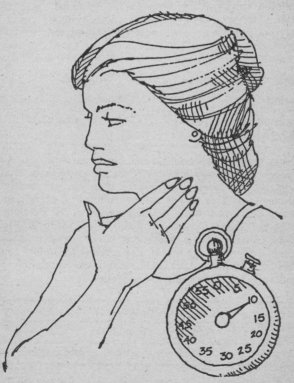

Count your pulse rate by gently pressing your fingers against the artery located approximately two inches to the left of your windpipe.

two hours of tennis. And twenty minutes on a bicycle, maintaining a speed of twenty miles per hour (not fast) provides you with more aerobic benefits than eighteen holes of golf.

In terms of aerobic benefits, the best forms of exercise are as follows:

OUTDOORS	INDOORS
1. Jogging (walking briskly is nearly as good)	1. Running in place
2. Bicycling	2. Jumping rope
3. Swimming	3. Stationary bike
4. Cross-country skiing	4. Rowing machine
5. Skating	5. Treadmill
6. Vigorous handball, basketball, racquet ball	6. "Aerobic dance"

Twenty seems to be a magic number in aerobics. Most experts agree that twenty minutes of steady exercise is what it takes to get your body working so that you are receiving aerobic benefits. This means twenty minutes of exercising so that your heart is beating at no lower than 70 percent or higher than 85 percent of your maximum output level. That's 70 to 85 percent of the maximum heart rate that doctors recommend for your age group. For a reference point, take a look at the following chart of minimum and maximum output levels arranged according to age groups.

Heart Rates for Aerobic Benefits		
Age	Heartbeats per minute	
	Minimum (70%)	Maximum (85%)
20-25	140	167
26-30	134	163
31-35	131	159
36-40	127	155

41-45	124	150
46-50	120	146
51-55	117	142
56-60	113	138
61-65	110	133
66-70	106	129

If you do not like keeping track of things by number, you may prefer this method. Exercise at the maximum level you can while still being able to carry on a conversation with a friend. If you're running alone, try singing a song while you're running. The conversation or song can come out jerky and offbeat, that's okay. But when it becomes difficult to converse or sing, slow down.

Minimum exercise programs as recommended by Dr. Kenneth Cooper look something like this:

Running:	6 miles per week
Biking:	30 miles per week
Swimming:	1.5 miles per week
Walking:	15 miles per week

Each time you exercise, give yourself a fifteen-minute warm-up period. Gentle stretching exercises are especially important for runners. Such things as touching your toes and doing sit-ups are good, if you remember to stretch *easily* and *gently*, never bouncing or forcing your muscles. *Runner's Handbook*, published by Penguin Books, New York, is an excellent reference for stretching exercises, both for conditioning muscles unaccustomed to running and for helping to prevent specific kinds of runner's injuries. A similar book for the bicyclist is *John Marino's Bicycling Book*, published by J. P. Tarcher, for which I am a co-author with John Marino, who holds the world's record for cycling from Los Angeles to Manhattan.

After a good run, always give yourself a cooling-off period. This allows your heart and lungs to gently return to their normal operating rates. To cool off, simply plan on walking, rather than running, that last few hundred feet home. Let your heart rate return to about 110 beats per minute or less before you go in to sit down.

FURTHER READING

Bicycling Magazine (monthly publication). Emmaus, Pa.: Rodale Press.

Cooper, Kenneth H. *New Aerobics*. New York: M. Evans, 1970.

Fixx, James F. *The Complete Book of Running*. New York: Random House, 1977.

Higdon, Hal. *Fitness After Forty*. Mountain View, Ca.: World Publications, 1977.

Marino, John; May, L., M.D.; and Bennett, Hal. *John Marino's Bicycling Book*. Los Angeles, Ca.: J. P. Tarcher, 1981.

Runner's World (monthly publication). Runner's World, Inc., Box 36, Mountain View, Ca. 94042.

Ullyot, Joan. *Women's Running*. Mountain View, Ca.: World Publications, 1977.

8.

Fueling the Doctor Within: The Role of Nutrition in Health

TRADITIONAL MEDICINE HAS, until very recently, ignored the role of nutrition in health. Although quite a bit of skepticism still prevails, especially where fad diets and megavitamin therapies are concerned, physicians are definitely taking a more thoughtful look at diet these days.

Many of the positive aspects of diet they are discovering will seem obvious to those of us who are conscious of what we eat. The rationale in support of eating well is as simple as the fact that *a good diet feels good*. You feel satisfied and content after eating, not distressed and slightly anxious about your symptoms of indigestion. Feeling good, feeling relaxed and satisfied, represents a mental and physical state that benefits the doctor within, in much the same way that deep relaxation does.

There was a time in our parents' and grandparents' lives

when many of the wisdoms we are now discovering were second nature. People knew their food sources, even down to the names of the farmers who supplied the apples they ate and the milk their children drank. One could judge what he was getting by driving past the land where the food was grown or the cattle grazed. One also knew the reputations of the families who supplied the food.

What a contrast those days were to our present life-style, when our food sometimes comes from hundreds, or even thousands of miles away! Even when fresh fruits are in season and grown nearby, the produce we buy at the supermarket may come from distant sources or it may be last year's crop which has been kept in cold storage. Why is all this important? It's important because both transporting and storing food reduces its nutritional values. In addition, many of our foods are now processed, with nonfood substances added for color or prolonged shelf life, or flavor. Often these nonfood substances have names we can't even pronounce. Consider the following:

- Dr. Roger J. Williams, who discovered the important B vitamin pantothenic acid, and who was the director of the Clayton Foundation Biochemical Institute (University of Texas), put laboratory rats on a diet of good old-fashioned American enriched white bread. After ninety days, two-thirds of the rats were dead. The surviving third were suffering from severe malnutrition and stunted growth.

- Dr. Donald R. Davis, at the University of California at Irvine, put rats on a regimen modeled after the typical American diet. It included: bread (white, enriched), sugar, eggs, milk, ground beef, cabbage, potatoes, tomatoes, oranges, apples, bananas, and coffee. Compared to another group of rats that was fed on Purina Rat Chow, the rats on the American diet fell far behind in growth rates and general health.

- Junk foods (foods with few or no nutrients) now account for 26 percent of the average caloric intake in the United States. Similarly, on the average, the American gets 45 percent of his calories from refined carbohydrate products rather than from whole or nonmanufactured food sources.

• Dr. Carl C. Pfeiffer,* of the Brain Bio Center in Princeton, New Jersey, shows in his research that between 2,500 and 3,000 different kinds of food additives are in use today. What is more alarming is that the average consumer ingests five pounds of these additives per year!

In many cases, the aches and pains we have, the everyday stresses of minor indigestion, or low energy, or depression, or vulnerability to infection, or allergic reactions, or lack of ability to concentrate, or even hyperactivity in children can be traced to the things we eat. Your doctor within is powerful, but without certain micronutrients (vitamins and minerals) he can't work to full potential. Furthermore, bombarded by chemicals such as food coloring derived from petroleum by-products, or sodium nitrites, and a multitude of other laboratory inventions ingested through our foods, the doctor within can be doubly handicapped.

In 1975, Ben F. Feingold, M.D., published a book called *Why Your Child is Hyperactive,*† which was based on his experiences as the chief of the allergy department at the Kaiser-Permanente Medical Center in San Francisco. In his practice he worked with children whose allergies could not be traced to the usual allergens such as milk, chocolate, wheat, eggs, cheese, and cola drinks. He found that by taking these children off junk foods—food products that contained artificial flavoring and coloring—symptoms such as skin allergies and hyperactivity disappeared. Although the main part of his work was with children, there were adults in the study who responded similarly.

Since the publication of his book, a group by the name of the Nutrition Foundation has published tests they have done that would seem to refute Dr. Feingold's studies. It is interesting to note, however, that this scientific group, the Nutrition Foundation, was established and is funded by the Coca-Cola company, the Life Savers company, and several other giant manufacturers of processed foods and snacks.

---

* Dr. Carl C. Pfeiffer, *Mental and Elemental Nutrients: A Physician's Guide to Nutrition and Health Care* (New Canaan, Conn.: Keats Publishing, Inc., 1976).

† Ben F. Feingold, *Why Your Child Is Hyperactive* (New York: Bantam Books, 1976).

Before I describe the positive steps you might take to improve your diet, I think it's important to know the harmful effects of many of the ingredients in the foods you probably eat.

Refined flours. Used in most snack foods and a great number of breads, these flours have been associated with a wide variety of diseases, ranging from indigestion to constipation to hypoglycemia and the inability to concentrate. Lack of bulk in refined flours is the main culprit in these digestion problems, while lack of the B vitamins, removed in the refining processes, may be the cause of the mental dysfunctions that seem to go along with this product.

Sugar. It is shocking to learn that the average American consumes over 100 pounds of sugar per year. This figure includes sugar used in the processing of beer, wine, and other alcoholic beverages; the sugar coating on cereals; sugar added to cereals other than the sugar-coated ones; sugar added to canned fruits, bread, and meats in fast food such as hamburgers; even sugar added to peanut butter. In addition, there's the sugar we add to our coffee or tea, the sugar we sprinkle on our cornflakes, the sugar in that midmorning pastry, the sugar in cola drinks, cookies, pies, chewing gum, ice cream, candy bars, and even salted peanuts. When you stop to consider that refined sugar, derived by processing sugar beets, was invented in 1801, and that refined sugar satisfies no nutritional needs, there can be little argument that our national *sweet tooth* is an acquired habit. It may be true that sugar tastes good and gives you quick energy, but as the day wears on sugar intake decreases your level of energy. The result, for most people, is a vague feeling of depression and tension, and even a headache.

Fats. Doctors are also paying attention to the fat content in our diets. The subject of cholesterol promises much in the treatment and prevention of heart disease. Laboratory findings have supported medical statistics in the view that high fat intake overtaxes the doctor within. A kind of plaque builds up within our artery walls as the result of high-fat diets, and the doctor within can't clear it. This plaque, unless the diet is changed, continues to build up, hardening the arteries, destroying their usual elasticity. The result? The arteries break down, no longer capable of feeding blood to the heart. In simple, everyday terms, this is a heart attack.

The fat content of the foods you eat has a very clear-cut effect on the flow of lymph in your body. Because your lymph system cooperates with your digestive system in processing fats, a meal with high fat content will make your lymph fluid become thick and milky. Physiologists tell us that it can be as much as 2 percent fat. The fluid will move sluggishly as a result.

Not only eating fats but storing them in your body increases the amount of fat that will be in both your lymph and blood. So, in addition to cutting down on fats in your diet, weight management can be an asset to keeping your lymph system working well.

Salt. It is estimated that the average American consumes approximately one tablespoon of salt per day, which is twelve times as much salt as he needs. This causes his tissues to retain too much water. The release of fluid in your body is normal. It is the source of fluid surrounding every cell, and it is the source of fluid in your lymph system. Both the lymph and the blood are influenced by fluid balances in your body and impaired when too much fluid is retained. In most climates, and for most people, a salt intake of about one gram (.035 ounce) a day is sufficient.

Diuretics. These are chemicals that cause your body to excrete fluids. Dehydration and mineral imbalances, which can result from a reduction in fluid, will have a potentially damaging effect on the lymph system. Diuretic tablets are often prescribed for people with high blood pressure, who retain too much fluid, but most of us should avoid chemicals with a diuretic effect. These are contained in coffee, tea, cola drinks, and caffeine drinks. Alcohol is also diuretic. Interestingly enough, caffeine and alcohol drinks also bring about an increase in the amount of fat in your circulatory system.

Diet as a Remedy for Indigestion, Constipation, and Serious Gastrointestinal Diseases

One of the first food theories to be widely accepted by the medical community in recent years was the idea of introducing more bulk into the average American's diet. Medical statistics show a marked increase in gastrointestinal diseases as bulk is reduced in the everyday diet. Bulk is the roughage in vegetables and grains, the indigestible part of the food that is broken down, refined out, in our processed foods.

The intestines are well served by the doctor within, but the movement of stool through these muscular channels requires a particular relationship between the organ and its contents. Low bulk slows the movement. High bulk moves it along. This becomes important when you learn that normal stool contains substances that are carcinogenic. These carcinogens pose no threat to the bowel if stool movement is rapid. It is only when the stool rests for long periods in our bodies that these carcinogens threaten us. Thus, high bulk, by keeping the stool moving at the rate it should, minimizes the threat of cancer of the colon.

Low-bulk diets also produce constipation. And with constipation comes straining to evacuate the contents of one's bowels. This straining produces a pressure in blood veins, causing varicose veins in the legs and hemorrhoids in the rectum. Some physicians even speculate that venous pressures caused by straining at the toilet may also contribute to heart disease.

If you're eating well you should have no need whatsoever for antacids or laxatives, at least not on a regular basis. Occasionally, during periods of high stress, overwork, or perhaps while traveling, indigestion or constipation can occur and you might be tempted to seek relief in such remedies. But if you are using these remedies regularly, and your physician tells you you're otherwise healthy, you are definitely overtaxing your doctor within.

In the first place, medical studies tell us that antacids don't work for most people. This inclues all the popular preparations containing one or more of the following: aluminum hydroxide, magnesium, and sodium bicarbonate. Antacids with algin, which coats the stomach with a thick, gel-like substance, do seem to bring some relief for some people. However, antacid use is definitely unhealthy, since it affects the ability of your digestive system to absorb certain micronutrients. Continuous antacid use can deplete your system of calcium, making your bones porous and brittle. This demineralization process can be the cause of "bone pain" and even osteoporosis, a crippling disease.

Maintaining calcium is important not only because it is one of the minerals (electrolytes) that spark the communication of nerve cells but also because a good warehouse of calcium prevents our bodies from taking up strontium 90, a by-product of all nuclear reactions, both man-made and natural. Once in our bones, strontium 90 can destroy the genetic material of normal body cells and cause them to go wild, that is, to become malignant and cause tumors.

Remember, vitamins K and the B complex are produced in your intestines, and these important tools of your doctor within can be reduced or weakened through the use of laxatives or antacids. If you are troubled by indigestion or constipation, first look to changes in your diet for relief. Eat more raw foods, which have more bulk and aid the digestive processes. Also eat whole cereal products, such as health food store granola, breads made of whole grains, and unprocessed rice or bulgur instead of fried or processed mashed potatoes.

Exercise is also a great aid to digestion. Having a leisurely walk after your evening meal not only aids digestion, essentially through a kind of massaging action that this provides for your intestines, but it also helps you relax and sleep. A leisurely walk of a mile a day is excellent for this.

Are you a person who spends all your time on your feet, who is constantly on the run? I know this sounds like a contradiction, but you, especially, can benefit from this evening walk. The leisurely aspect of this exercise allows you to relax muscles that more purposeful, work-related physical activity has tightened and stiffened. Try it for ten days and see if you don't benefit greatly.

Digestive problems can be easily avoided. The message

should be clear: Understand that the discomfort you feel after eating is a message from your body telling you that it can't handle what you've just done to it. If you are a normal, healthy person you should feel complete comfort after eating. If you don't, you need to start changing your dietary habits. Whatever you do, never complicate your condition by adding still another chemical insult to your doctor within.

Easy Changes for a Healthier Diet

To provide your doctor within with everything needed to keep you healthy, start changing your diet in small steps.

When you shop at the supermarket, pass up the baked goods, canned goods, frozen goods, soda pop, salted snacks, and deli counter. Spend your time at the meat counter, dairy counter, and fresh produce section. Seek new recipes for cheese and dairy products, both for nutrition and to save money on your meat budget. Avoid preserved meat products, since most of these are high in nitrites.

For breakfast cut out all sugar-coated cereals. Substitute plain yogurt topped with fruit and a couple of heaping tablespoonfuls of granola. I am not recommending the kind of granola that is beautifully packaged and expensively promoted in the supermarket. You'll discover upon reading the labels that most of that stuff is packed with sugar, in some cases even more sugar than sugar-frosted cornflakes or wheat puffs. What you want is the kind of granola that is sold in health food stores, frequently in simple plastic bags, and which is not loaded with sugar.

If you like eggs for breakfast, cook them with minimum amounts of oils or animal fats. Try eggs poached, boiled, or lightly scrambled with only enough oil to season the pan. Bacon lovers take heed! Health food stores and a few supermarkets are beginning to carry bacon and sausage without nitrites. Read package labels carefully, and look for the nitrite-free products in the frozen food section.

If you're accustomed to having a piece of pastry with coffee for a midmorning snack, substitute an apple, orange, or other piece of fruit. Or try a cup of plain yogurt or cottage cheese with fresh fruit slices. (Avoid flavored yogurts, sold in many supermarkets, which can be as high in sugar as a Danish pastry.) You may find that the Continental custom of a piece of fruit and a slice of cheese is far more satisfying than a puffed pastry with sugar frosting and a cup of coffee.

For lunches look on the restaurant menu for some of the new vegetarian and cheese sandwiches that are becoming so popular. Substitute these, now and then, for hamburgers, cold cuts, or a BLT.

When you sit down to eat, *start* at least one meal per day with a large salad. Make salads with a variety of vegetables; try fresh spinach leaves in addition to or instead of lettuce. Have chopped celery, onions, radishes, tomatoes, carrots, even apple, raw mushrooms, and raw, sliced zucchini or summer squash in your salads. Try adding crisp, fresh sprouts, and sunflower seeds for variety. Make your own salad dressings, light on the oil, mixed with apple cider vinegar rather than wine vinegar, which tends to leach vitamin C. Use lemon juice and herbs for extra flavor. A thick creamy salad dressing can be made quickly and easily by mixing (for each serving) a heaping tablespoon of plain yogurt with a teaspoon of mayonnaise, a shot of fresh garlic, a sprinkle of basil and a dash of freshly ground pepper.

Fill up on salad *before* the main course. You'll soon find yourself cutting back on your meat portions, but enjoying what you do eat more than ever. Since you've already eaten all the vegetables you need in the salad, you can leave the traditional cooked vegetable off the main course platter. A small baked potato with yogurt and chopped chives becomes a delicious, healthful replacement for a butter-, gravy-, or sour cream-drenched potato.

Instead of salt, try putting a cellar of mixed ground herbs on the table. Herbs such as oregano, basil, thyme, and dill are the *secret* ingredients of some of the world's most delicious sauces. Experiment with your own mixtures until you find something that you like.

Avoid most salt substitutes, which may be more harmful than the thing they're designed to replace. Monosodium glutamate (MSG), not a substitute in itself, is sometimes used to pep up seasonings sold to replace salt. But MSG has side effects that include a burning sensation throughout your body, headache, nausea, and extreme thirst. Not everyone seems to be sensitive to this drug, but it is a frequent enough complaint that every hospital emergency room sees its share of patients with Chinese Restaurant Syndrome.* MSG is a sodium, and it does cause retention of water just as salt does, but its flavor-enhancing capacities are greater than those of salt. For this reason, smaller quantities are needed to get extra flavor, and so can be mixed with salt or low-sodium preparations to encourage less intake of salt.

Salt substitutes using potassium chloride do not have the side effects of substitutes containing MSG. Adelle Davis used to recommend mixing potassium chloride with regular iodized salt for the table.† But again, read labels. In a recent trip to the supermarket I discovered two brands of potassium chloride salt substitute with MSG added.

Most doctors tell us that we should be drinking somewhere between six and ten glasses of water per day. This includes the water we take in with coffee, juices, tea, and soft drinks. If you're exercising each day, your ideal fluid intake may be considerably more. For those who exercise regularly, the sensation of thirst is an accurate indicator of need. Frequently, people who do not exercise regularly do not consume enough water, and they sometimes mistake thirst for hunger, satisfying the latter when the former is what their body is indicating.

Hot weather, your individual chemistry, and stress can cause you to need more fluids, as can the fever that comes with an infection. It is particularly important when you have an infection to keep your lymph system working well. But often, when you're ill, you feel neither hungry nor thirsty. At such times, it is good to remind yourself to keep up your fluid intake, because it helps keep the lymph system active.

Try herb teas to replace caffeine drinks. And if you must drink soft drinks pick one that isn't a cola. There are many delicious herb teas on the shelves of the supermarkets

---

* See "Chinese Restaurant Syndrome," *The Merck Manual,* 13th ed. (Rahway, N.J.: Merck & Co., Inc., 1977), p. 798.

† Adelle Davis, *Let's Get Well* (New York: New American Library, 1972).

nowadays, and you're sure to find one that will satisfy your palate.

REDUCING FATS IN YOUR DIET

As general guidelines for cutting down on fats and improving your health, keep the following points in mind:

1. Trim fat from raw meat. Then broil, roast, or boil the meat instead of frying it.
2. Eat foods other than meat and eggs for breakfast and lunch whenever you can—cereals for breakfast, vegetarian sandwiches or salads for lunch.
3. Eat beef or pork no more than three times a week. If you must have meat, have fish or fowl. Remove the skin from fowl, since it is high in fat. Look into Chinese, Mexican, and Turkish cookbooks for delicious vegetarian alternatives.
4. Cook with a good quality olive oil or other vegetable oils, rather than with lard.
5. Dairy products are also high in animal fats. Reduce your intake of whole milk, cheese, butter, sour cream, whipped cream, and ice cream. Substitute low-fat milk, buttermilk, yogurt, soft margarine, and cottage cheese.

Diet changes come slowly. Tastes are learned, supported by years of habit. But recognize that new tastes do develop. It just takes time. Make small changes initially. These small changes will accumulate until there will come a day when you suddenly realize you're enjoying a completely different fare than you did a few months before. You'll feel healthier, you'll have more energy, and you'll be giving your doctor within all the stuff needed for creating health.

LOSING WEIGHT

Obesity, or overweight, either aggravates or causes a long list of diseases, ranging from high blood pressure to stroke and heart attack to musculoskeletal disorders to diabetes to lowered self-esteem. Most experts agree that there would be at least a 25 percent decrease in heart disease among people under sixty-five through dietary changes alone.

Most average Americans can lose weight simply by cutting all sugared foods from their diets, substituting only solidly nutritional ones. But sugar, like salt, isn't easy to ignore. It beckons us like a Siren's song. The more you use it, the more you want it. And, what's worse, sugar, like salt, excites your taste buds and stimulates your appetite. If you could stop your intake of sugar and salt you'd find that your desire for food would diminish, and that you would eat something closer to what your body *needed* rather than *wanted*.

Most overweight people eat when they are anxious or under pressure. And because most snack foods are sugary and/or salty, the desire for food is further exaggerated. Substituting low caloric foods for other snacks is a powerful aid in breaking this cycle. Eat apples, oranges, celery, or carrots for snacks. Keep them handy, at home and on the job, so that whenever you reach for a quick snack you won't have to hunt for a more fattening alternative.

Another factor contributing to overweight is "unconscious eating." When eating under pressure, most people don't taste their food and so come to the end of a meal unsatisfied, feeling they still have to eat. While watching television or when you're involved in an engrossing conversation you might also eat unconsciously. Your mind focuses on the television program or on the conversation instead of the experience of eating. The nerves of your taste buds get shut down or short-circuited, and after you've finished eating you still have not had the *experience* of eating. You may be able to control your food intake better simply by paying attention to your food. Enjoy the sensual experience of eating, which is nearly as necessary as ingesting the nutrients themselves.

Avoid eating before going to bed. Not only does this food habit put on extra pounds, but it can also disturb your sleep, keeping your stomach working long after it should be at rest. A leisurely walk an hour before going to bed at night helps you digest your food, burn up calories, and helps your body prepare both emotionally and physiologically for sleep. And don't forget that this exercise also gets your lymph system moving.

In his book, *The American Way of Life,** John W. Farquhar, M.D., provides some important tools for reducing. He bases his weight reduction plan on the theory that food habits are learned. Losing weight should be approached as a permanent habit change. That is, improve your daily food habits forever. Avoid the slim-to-fat cycle, the fad diet route, which is hard on your body. The following suggestions should help.

THE THREE PRINCIPLES OF PERMANENT WEIGHT CONTROL

1. Become aware of your present eating habits by writing down everything you eat in a day. Record the time of day you eat, when you eat, and what else you are doing while you eat. Keep these records for a week or so before you start any changes in your diet. They will tell you a lot about your present eating habits.

2. Learn about food. What kinds are nutritious while being low in calories? What kinds are best for your digestive system? What kinds of foods satisfy you while not teasing you into eating too much?

3. Incorporate new foods into your diet slowly, until you have cut empty calories and unconscious eating down to a minimum.

What is your ideal weight? Dr. Farquhar provides this simple formula:

- *For men:* Multiply your height in inches by 4. Subtract 128 from this total. That's your ideal weight, in the nude.
- *For women:* Multiply your height in inches by 3.5 Subtract 108 from this total. That's your ideal weight, in the nude.

These are ideal weights for people of average build. However, if you're a delicate-boned and small-muscled person,

---

* John W. Farquhar, *The American Way of Life Need Not Be Hazardous to Your Health* (New York: Norton, 1979).

you may find these numbers too high. If you're big-boned and muscular you may find them too low. Add or subtract a few pounds if you're at these extremes.

Vitamins as an Aid to the Doctor Within

Even the best vitamin pills in the world won't replace eating good-quality food, but there are times when vitamins can be helpful. Those times are when, for one reason or another, you feel your present diet is lacking, when you are under stress, when you are ill, when you are getting more physical exercise than usual, and in the winter months when we are naturally eating fewer fresh foods, that is, foods with fewer nutrients.

Nutritionists generally agree that most severe vitamin deficiencies will handicap antibody production and slow down the repair of tissue damaged by disease or trauma. Vitamins A, the B complex, and C, along with bioflavonoids, are the ones best known for their ability to help your body resist infection and restore health after illness.

Three other vitamins are known to be directly associated with antibody and white blood cell production and activity. These are choline, folic acid, and pantothenic acid. Brewer's yeast, wheat germ, green leafy vegetables, legumes, organ meats, egg yolks, and whole grains all contain large quantities of all these essential antibody vitamins.

All three of these vitamins should be taken together if possible, since each helps your body absorb the others. B complex and C vitamins also help in the absorption of these vitamins. Sugar, alcohol, caffeine, and stress, on the other hand, reduce your ability to absorb choline, folic acid, and pantothenic acid.

Since brewer's yeast contains all three of these vitamins, along with others that help in their absorption, that's probably the single best food for assuring yourself of antibody production. One or two tablespoons of brewer's yeast taken with orange juice, yogurt, or whole grain breakfast cereals provides you with a sufficient source of these vitamins.

Occasionally, in some people, large quantities of brewer's

yeast cause gas. If this happens, reduce your intake to about two teaspoons per day, then increase it gradually to a level your body will easily tolerate.

If you're eating plenty of fresh, leafy green vegetables each day, and you aren't taking in large quantities of sugar, caffeine, or alcohol, the chances are good that you are getting sufficient quantities of these "antibody-building" vitamins.

If you are taking a vitamin-mineral supplement, read the label to see what you're getting. You should be getting a minimum of 1 milligram of folic acid, 10 milligrams of pantothenic acid. There are no USDA standards established for choline, but nutritionists' estimates place it at about the same as you'd get with the yolk of a single egg; that would be a minimum of 250 milligrams.

On a daily basis, vitamin B_{12} is essential in the production of RNA and DNA, the genetic material of your cells, which are reproducing twenty-four hours a day. This vitamin is then directly used by your doctor within to rebuild damaged tissue. Tolerance for stress is also heightened by maintaining a good intake of B_{12}. It is important to note here that the consumption of refined sugar drains the body's stores of this vitamin.

Sleep, that important period of your life during which your doctor within does so much work, can also be affected by diet. Most people know how indigestion can interrupt their sleep. Beyond that, we know that vitamin C, inositol, and B_6 intake can mean the difference between sleeping well and not sleeping at all.

Vitamins A, D, and E are used in the maintenance of healthy skin and blood vessels. Electrolytes, minerals such as calcium and magnesium, maintain the minute electrical charges in each of your cells, in the absence of which there would be no life. Many other vitamins, minerals, and trace elements play important roles in metabolizing fats and carbohydrates. Still others are necessary in allowing your body to absorb other micronutrients. For example, vitamin C is necessary in absorbing iron, which prevents anemia.

Research indicates that a number of vitamins and minerals that help our bodies regulate cholesterol also aid your doctor within in handling stress adequately.

VITAMINS TO TAKE IN TIMES OF STRESS

1. The B vitamins, notably B_3 (niacin), B_6 (pyridoxine), folic acid (folacin), and B_{12}: Help the body digest or get rid of extra cholesterol.

2. Vitamin C: Research demonstrates that it can lower blood cholesterol levels,* and strengthen blood vessels.

3. Vitamin E: Thought to prevent oxidation of fatty acids that can cause plaque in arteries.

4. Magnesium, potassium, manganese, vanadium, selenium, and zinc:† Promote enzyme activities, stimulate hormone production, help in processing of fats and carbohydrates.

5. Choline, biotin, lecithin, B_{15} (pangamic acid), and inositol: Prevent accumulation of fat in the liver.‡

Most health food stores, and an increasing number of drugstores, carry balanced formulas of vitamin/mineral capsules that will provide most of these nutrients at levels that will benefit you. Buy formulas with everything you need in one pill; don't attempt to purchase a whole armful of separate bottles of pills. For one thing, the balanced formula gives you some assurance that you won't be getting too much of one nutrient and not enough of another. A good balanced formula, one in which all the supplements you need come in one pill, is far less expensive than buying the separate nutrients.

As a general guideline for buying vitamin/mineral supplements in balanced formulas, I use the following amounts. However, if you are taking any kind of medication, especially if you are taking diuretics, or if you are on a physician-directed diet, consult with your doctor before taking vitamin supplements.

---

* C. Spittle, "Atherosclerosis and Vitamin C," *Lancet*, December 11, 1971.

† Carl C. Pfeiffer, *Mental and Elemental Nutrients* (New Canaan, Conn.: Keats Publishing, Inc., 1975).

‡ Ibid.

RECOMMENDED DAILY ALLOWANCES OF VITAMINS, MINERALS, AND TRACE ELEMENTS

(Look for a supplement formula with all or most of these in a single pill.)

Vitamins
A—10,000 I.U.
D—400 I.U.
E—50 I.U.
C—500 mg.
Folic Acid—0.1 mg.
B_1—5 mg.
B_2—5 mg.
Niacinamide—50 mg.
B_6—10 mg.
B_{12}—10 mcg.
Biotin—10 mcg.
Pantothenic acid—50 mg.
Choline—20 mg.

Minerals
Calcium—100 mg.
Phosphorus—20 mg.
Iodine—100 mcg.
Iron—20 mg.
Magnesium—100 mg.
Copper—0.5 mg.
Zinc—20 mg.
Manganese—5 mg.
Potassium—10 mg.

Trace Elements
PABA—100 mg.
Bioflavonoids—25 mg.

FURTHER READING

Dinaberg, Kathy, and Akel, D'Ann. *Nutrition Survival Kit.* San Francisco: Panjandrum Press, 1976.

Lappé, Frances Moore. *Diet for a Small Planet.* New York: Ballantine, 1975.

Pfeiffer, Carl C. *Mental and Elemental Nutrients.* New Canaan, Conn.: Keats Publishing, Inc., 1975.

Robertson, Flinders, and Godfrey. *Laurel's Kitchen.* New York: Bantam Books, 1978.

Williams, Dr. Roger J. *Nutrition Against Disease.* New York: Bantam Books, 1973.

Epilogue

IN AN IDEAL FUTURE WORLD, modern medicine will offer freedom from disease that we of our generation can only imagine. Advances made in our own lifetimes, in fields such as miniaturized electronics and computers, suggest that organs and limbs (and even eyes), damaged through disease or accident, may one day be replaced by counterparts made in factories. Indeed, we already replace hip, knee, and elbow joints with plastics. Portions of blood vessels can be replaced with synthetic counterparts, while "pacemakers" electronically stimulate heart contractions to correct certain kinds of heart disease. Chronic, debilitating pain can now be controlled with brain implants through which a person can block pain impulses by pushing a button. Scientists tell us that in the next ten years there will be electronic glasses to provide sight to the blind.

If I were a science fiction writer, it might be fun to take all this a step further, into the field of disease prevention. The technology is evolving, for example, that will one day allow us to implant microscopic sensors in a person's body at birth. These sensors could monitor the state of that person's health every moment of the day. Signals from the sensors would be communicated to central computers in each of the major cities, computers that had access to all the medical knowledge available in the world. These computers would analyze complex signals from the human body and compare them with optimal health standards stored in electronic memory banks. Whenever less than optimal health was indicated in any individual, this information would be communicated to a laboratory close by. The lab would analyze the problem, synthesize medication to restore optimal health, and deliver treatment to the person in need within a matter of minutes. We would then have created an electronic doctor within.

Sounds fantastic. Such a system would require an investment of billions of dollars, with computer problems that might take decades just to program. Theoretically, the technology to accomplish all this is within our reach. However, the system still has one glaring fault: Its capabilities would be limited by the knowledge medical scientists possess about the human body and health. Like everything else in computer science, the machinery is only as good as the human minds that create it.

The electronic doctor within would have to *understand* infinitely more than all our medical scientists presently do. It would have to monitor early signals of disease that no one has yet identified. It would have to be capable of producing miracle drugs that are presently beyond the grasp of our most gifted biochemists.

But before getting carried away with our own brilliance, let's stop and take a look around. The fact of the matter is that our utopian system of health already exists. It exists within every human body. And the full capacities of this system are already quite beyond the grasp of the world's most advanced medical scientists. The power that each of us has within us to prevent illness and to heal and restore tissue damaged by illness or accident far surpasses anything existing even in the most advanced medical centers. At its very best, medical science can *aid* these inner healing capacities, but without them nothing medical science has to offer could bring normal, lasting health.

The Activated Patient

A new term is beginning to make its way into our society. It is "the activated patient," and it refers to people who are taking active roles in their own health care. If you have ever asked your doctor to explain a treatment he or she has prescribed for you, you are an activated patient. If you have ever asked for a second opinion on a medical decision, you are an activated patient. The fact that you are now reading this book is good evidence that you are, or want to be, an activated patient.

As an increasing number of people gain information about what they can do to be healthy, doctors find they can spend less time on "invasive" treatments, such as drugs and surgery, and more time on patient education. But in order for this trend to continue both patients and doctors must change. First, patients must seek out medical information to guide them in choices they can make for health. And second, doctors must be willing to seek ways to communicate more information to their patients. Where the physician must give up traditional authority roles, the patient must be willing to face the fact that doctors alone can't heal.

We do have a choice about health. Learning both about our bodies and the limits of modern medicine puts each of us in a more powerful position of control than we have ever enjoyed in history.

As our knowledge of disease and health grows, we expand our range of choices. Health becomes less a matter of chance or fate and more a matter of individual volition. We should celebrate the fact that knowledge gleaned from the most sophisticated medical research, research that was previously accessible only to doctors, is now available to all of us, presented in popular books, television programs, and classes that require no previous medical training to understand. The knowledge is available for us to have mastery over most of the diseases that presently trouble us, but taking the next step is not the physician's responsibility: It is the patient's.

In an ideal future world the physician will be a teacher and counselor rather than a dispenser of pills and a manipulator of the scalpel. And we, the patients, no longer satisfied with making high priests of our physicians, will establish open partnerships with the medical community, with our mutual goal being the creation of health. Patient and physician will join with the doctor within, who over the past two billion years has developed greater healing powers than we can imagine even in our wildest dreams.

Index

Activated patient, concept of, 139–40
Acupressure, for headache relief, 89–90
Acupuncture, 87, 89
Adenoviruses, 11
Adrenal glands, 100, 110–11
stress and, 68–70
Air conditioning, infections and, 16
Alcohol, 104, 122, 123, 132
Allergies, 23, 121
Alveoli, 15–16
Amantadine, 46
American Association for the Advancement of Tension, 98
American Association for the Study of Headache, 98
American Cancer Society, 45
American Way of Life, The (Farquhar), 131
Anemia, 17, 133
Angina, 97
Annals of Internal Medicine, 5–6
Antacids, 124–25

Antibiotics, 1, 5
effective use of, 22–23
interferon compared to, 44–45
pros and cons of, 17, 19–22
types of resistance to, 21
Antibodies, 7, 9–10, 18, 30, 34–38
exercise for strengthening of, 110–11
stress and, 68–69, 70–71, 111
time needed for formation of, 37–38
vitamins and, 132–33
Antigens, 34–36, 38, 39
vaccinations and, 39–40
Antiperspirants, 24–25
Antipyretic medication, 28
Archives of General Psychiatry, 102
Arterial pulsation, lymph and, 53
Arteriosclerosis, 10
Arthritis, 3, 29
Arthritis Foundation, 97

More Reading from SIGNET and MENTOR

Buy them at your local

bookstore or use coupon

on next page for ordering.

SIGNET Books of Special Interest